THE POLITICS OF WESTERN MEDICINE

Papa Johnny's Book

Also by Holly Fourchalk

Adrenal Fatigue: Why am I so tired all the time?
Are you what you eat? Why Your Intestines Are the Foundation of Good Health
Cancer: Why what you don't know about your treatment could harm you.
Depression: The Real Cause May Be Your Body.
Diabetes: What Your Physician Doesn't Know
Glutathione: Your Body's Secret Healing Agent
Your Heart: Are you taking care of it?
Inflammation: The Silent Killer
Managing Your Weight: Why your body may be working against you and what you can do about it
The Chocolate Controversy: The Bad, the Mediocre and the Awesome
So What's the Point: If You Have Ever Asked
Your Immune System: Is Yours Protecting You?
Your Vital Liver: How to protect your liver from life's toxins

The Entwined Collection
Entwined: A Romantic Journey Back into Health
Entwined: The Ongoing Journey
Entwined: A Love that Crosses Time
Entwined: Arthritis: Manage It or Eliminate It
Entwined: When Is Enough Enough? (Coming Soon)

Tom's Collection
The Cosmic Socialite
Cosmic Healing
Cosmic Lessons
Cosmic Experience (Coming Soon)
Cosmic Choices (Coming Soon)
Continuing Journey (Coming Soon)

All of the above are available at DrHollyBooks.com

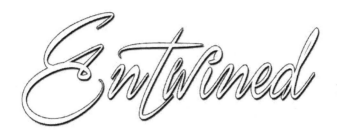

THE POLITICS OF WESTERN MEDICINE

Papa Johnny's Book

Holly Fourchalk

PhD., DNM®, RHT, AAP

Cover design by Peter Forde. Published by Vector Catalyst.

Choices Unlimited for Health & Wellness
Dr. Holly Fourchalk, Ph.D., DNM®, RHT, HT
Tel: 604.764.5203
Websites: www.ChoicesUnlimited.ca
         www.DrHollyBooks.com
E-mail: holly@choicesunlimited.ca

ISBN (softcover) 978-1-989420-06-5
ISBN (eBook) 978-1-989420-07-2

Disclaimer

This book is an attempt to increase awareness about health and the many options we have to bring the body back into a healthy balance.

Every effort has been made by the author, to ensure the information in this book is as accurate as possible. However, it is by no means a complete, or exhaustive, examination of all information.

The author believes in prevention and the superiority of a natural non-invasive approach to health over synthetic drugs and/or surgery.

As a Doctor of Natural Medicine, a researcher and teacher, the author knows what has worked for others and what worked for her. However, because our bodies are unique, any two individuals may experience different results from the same therapy. No two people are the same and the author cannot, and does not, render judgment or advice regarding a particular individual's situation.

The information collected within comes from a variety of researchers and sources from around the world who challenge the claims and politics of Conventional Western Medicine.

Research shows the top three leading causes of death in North America occurs directly from the physician/pharmaceutical component.

Repeatedly over the past several decades, we have witnessed claims and protocols determined by Western Conventional medicine to be more dangerous than beneficial.

Today ever-increasing numbers of people are aware of healing foods and herbs, supplements and modalities, but there are still far too many who are not. The fact that our physicians are part of this latter group makes healing even more challenging. Adding to this, another unfortunate fact is those who can profit from sickness and disease promote ignorance, creating devastating results.

It is the responsibility of the individual to find good professional health care practitioners to work with to resolve health issues and achieve optimal health.

To my Parents

For all their support and encouragement
My Dad for his ever-listening ear
My Mother for her open mind

Contents

Preface

Before we explore what The Entwined Collection is about, let's begin by understanding where Dr. Holly is coming from, and how and why she wants everyone to benefit.

Dr. Holly was born with a genetic disorder. Her delivery was a confusion of issues that went wrong; some of which were not recognized at the time. Her petite mal, or absence, seizures started when she was 4 years old, though nobody recognized what was happening. Absence seizures are named for the brief loss of consciousness, and often misinterpreted as daydreaming.

At the age of nine, she was in a dramatic accident which provoked, and accelerated, her female development. It also provoked the myoclonic seizures which manifested themselves in powerful twitches or muscle jerks or spasms. By the time she was 14, the petite mal seizures and myoclonic seizures now included grand mal, or tonic-clonic, seizures.

The grand mal/tonic-clonic seizures, a type of generalized seizure, affected the entire brain. During these types of seizures, she would lose consciousness and the skeletal muscles would thrash violently and uncontrollably followed by amnesia, headaches, a damaged tongue and exhaustion.

After Holly's first grand mal seizure, her mother found her passed out on the floor and was devastated. She had already lost two children; she was not prepared to lose another. The problem became more complex. The more medication Holly was put on, the more seizures she had; never mind all the weight and other issues the medications caused. Four, five, six mornings out of seven she woke up with petite mal and myoclonic seizures. The medical profession blamed the car accident and increased both the number of drugs and their dosage, which of course provoked more seizures.

Struggling to resolve the seizures, her mother attended medical conferences, even though she didn't understand half of what they were saying. She booked Holly into Naturopaths, Reflexologists, and Acupuncturists, and anyone who thought they could stop the seizures. They even worked with Edgar Cayce remedies. They had to find a way to stop the seizures.

It wasn't until Holly was studying neurological issues in university that she recognized she had been having seizures since she was four years old.

Holly's favorite and most beloved practitioner was Dr. Loffler, an Osteopath/Naturopath, whom she started to see at the age of 18. He identified a number of issues compounding the problem going back to the car accident. Her second favorite physician was the neurologist she started see at the age of 26. She identified the genetic issue that was causing the seizures and other problems. Holly learned that people with this type of disorder didn't usually graduate from high school and were usually dead by the time they were 26 years old. In addition, her EEGs indicated she shouldn't be able to talk.

In university she was diagnosed with an ovarian tumor the size of a hard ball. She was told she needed surgery immediately as it was dangerous. Dr. Loffler, however, put her on a specific diet for ovarian tumors. Due to family pressure, she underwent a second laparotomy 3.5 weeks later. The tumor was gone. Her medical doctors never asked how she accomplished that.

At the age of 26, she burnt her eyes and the specialist told her she had to join classes to learn how to be blind as she would be legally blind by the time she was 30. She went back a year and half later with 20/19 vision. He never asked how she accomplished that.

In school, Dr. Holly had to deal with issues like ADD (Attention Deficit Disorder) and Dyslexia, yet she studied hard and diligently and always maintained her honor roll marks. She loved numbers and went into university hoping to get degrees in Physics and Math and become an Astrophysicist. However, that wasn't the plan life had for her and she came out as a

Registered Psychologist. She ran her own practice for some 20 years.

During her training and practice as a psychologist, she was constantly frustrated at the total lack of training regarding the nutrients the brain required to function properly. Many of her clients came in with issues of depression and anxiety and other disorders. Dr. Holly would often suggest they see other practitioners like Naturopaths, Herbalists, or go for Hydro colonics. Repeatedly, supposed psychological issues were successfully solved, using other healing disciplines.

Dr. Holly attended Medical School as part of her of her first PhD, *PsychoNeuroEndocrinology*, which was in research and design. Two of the professors asked her to please stop asking questions. Why? Utilizing her knowledge in research and design; she repeatedly pointed out that referenced studies were not proving what they claimed. In fact, most of "evidenced based medicine" was not in fact, evidenced based – it was hypothesis based AND more and more of the hypotheses were being proven wrong. This was destroying the moral of the students.

Subsequently she learned how Big Pharma controls most Medical School Curriculums; and the Protocol and Procedure MDs are required to follow. In addition, they are now saying it can take up to 40 years for good research to get to the MDs and to the hospitals.

One thing Dr. Holly was never short on, was energy. Consequently, in addition to her academic profession and Psychology practice, Dr. Holly also opened and ran a big rig trucking company; an accounting business; a warehouse and distribution business and a rental company. However, she found herself challenged with the lack of morals and integrity in the trucking and warehousing businesses and eventually went back to school.

Dr. Holly got fed up with the limitations imposed on her within the field of psychology and enrolled in Naturopathic College. It was a double graduate program, 8 years completed in 4 years. Dr. Holly was also required to complete two years of Premed during the first year; meanwhile she continued her Psychology Practice.

By the time second year started, the seizures started up again. Very Scary. She hadn't had seizures for 15 years. In addition, other major health issues evolved. Her body kept telling her to quit. Holly was never a quitter. However, the College found out she was having seizures and put her on hold for a year. When she returned the following year, the seizures started up within three weeks, so she transferred from the Naturopathic program to a Doctor of Natural Medicine, wherein she could go at her own pace.

Holly went to India to complete, and intern for, for two Ayurveda medical programs. She also completed a

Masters in Herbal Medicine: *Bridging Ayurveda, Traditional Chinese Medicine and Western Herbal Medicine.* She studied homeopathy and reflexology, locally and abroad. She then applied and was accepted for a PhD program in Nutrition where she received a Cum Laude for her thesis identifying the biochemistry of cellular healing.

During this time, Dr. Holly applied to, and was accepted, into Law School. She wanted to know the ins and outs of law to protect practitioners from their Colleges and from Big Pharma.

While completing the various degrees, Dr. Holly worked with a mentor as she prepared to leave the College of Psychologists. In the meantime, the College of Psychologists accused her of practicing "non-evidence based' medicine. She volunteered to provide workshops teaching the nutrients that the brain required to function from a nutritional and biochemistry perspective, but they were not interested. She left.

Her practice as a Dr. of Natural Medicine was up and running by this time. She published twelve books for the general public over the next four years. She wanted the general public to understand the differences between Conventional Medicine/managing symptoms and REAL medicine/resolving the underlying issues.

The Entwined Collection

One day Dr. Holly woke up with an idea. Write a sexy romantic novel, that would attract a larger audience, incorporating a huge amount of health information explaining REAL medicine and *Entwined: A Romantic Journey Back into Health* came to fruition.

Preparing to go away on a vacation and write the sequel to *Entwined*, Dr. Holly woke up with the idea of the Round Table and asking each character in the book to write their own book. This way, she could a use all the different literary genres to convey a huge amount of information on health and wellness. People could enjoy learning about REAL health and medicine reading the writing genre they preferred: educational, romantic, mystery, political, etc. Consequently, each book in the Entwined Book Collection is written with a different slant and from a different perspective according to the character of the Entwined Book Project responsible for the book.

Dr. Holly attributes different healing disciplines to each of the Gibson family members who all work at the Gibson Clinic. With two exceptions: Dr. Holly is not a physiotherapist, and nor did she finish her Traditional Chinese Medicine program. Otherwise, Dr. Holly has all the degrees and designations to professionally address the issues focused on by her characters.

On a personal note, "**Entwined**" has a lot more meaning for Dr. Holly than just being the collection of books resulting from *Entwined: A Romantic Journey Back into Health*. The word Entwined reflects life itself. All aspects of our beingness are entwined: from the moral/ethical, to the spiritual/religious, to the intellectual/emotional, to the physical/sexual, to the family/social, to the ingestion/elimination, and to all the different energetics. They are all entwined. In addition, the individual is entwined with their family; with their social network; with the community; and with the nation. Again, all is entwined; encompassing the local to the universal. Nothing happens in isolation; entwined embraces all, whether local or all matter stretching throughout the universe.

Consequently, when we look at our health and wellbeing, we need to take the whole being into consideration. To isolate any aspect of our being, whether it be our physical health, psychological health, energetic health, etc. is to negate an aspect of who we are.

Two powerful words for Dr. Holly are **Entwined** and **Choices**. Just as our health is immeasurably entwined with all of whom we are; so are all our **choices entwined** with what we choose to do with those choices. Whether it is our symptoms, our health, our relationships, our careers, etc., we can choose to manage, or we can choose to eliminate. The **CHOICE** is ours.

All of us involved in the writing, editing, publishing and marketing of these books, hope you enjoy and learn a lot from the books. We wish you the very best of health.

Papa Johnny's Book

Papa Johnny was suffering from dementia. His physician prescribed him pharmaceuticals that were taking their toll on his health and his pocket book. Despite increasing dosages and adding more drugs, he was steadily going downhill.

Then his brother-in-law convinced him to go the Gibson Clinic and get real help.

He was able to get off the drugs, regain his mental capacity, and start living life again.

Papa Johnny was angry that he had gone through the mill with pharmaceuticals and started to do some research into both Western Conventional Medicine and "REAL" medicine.

The research resulted in this book, his contribution to the Entwined Collection.

Chapter 1
It all began when...

I am waiting patiently on the phone. This is going to be a big break for me. I get a real adrenaline rush when I uncover stories like this one. I have a passion for researching the underlying political and financial agendas and maneuvers.

I am retired now. I was a pretty healthy individual. Never suffered much in the way of ailments throughout my life.

I am not an academic but always prided myself on having a good mind. I loved to research and learn new things. I like to challenge concepts and play "devil's advocate" in debates. I certainly didn't waste my days in front a television or playing cards. I wasn't a dedicated athlete, but I did love to hike and bike ride and go for walks.

The past several years, however, have found me slowly retiring from life itself. I suffered from dementia – note I say suffered. Two reasons: one, I no longer suffer from dementia and two, dementia is not a physically painful issue – it is a mentally agonizing issue.

I was diagnosed with Alzheimer's which is one of many different types of dementia. Today they are realizing that mixed dementia is a lot more common than was previously recognized. In fact, the understanding of dementia is hugely changing. But there I was, taking more and more medications. The medications caused more problems and so they put me on even more medications.

I was virtually existing in front of the television. Why? The medications were obviously not resolving the problem; they were not even managing it. I was slowly dying. But then I found out, I didn't even have Alzheimer's and the type of dementia I had was reversible – and that is apparently not uncommon! I will share my story as I go along.

So, like I said, I get a real adrenaline rush when I get to uncover stories and help the public understand what is going on behind closed doors. Throughout life I have had an issue with people in power who take advantage of the rest of the population when they spew out misinformation, only provide some of the information, or mislead with false information.

I remember way back in my youth discussing morals, ethics and legalities with a lawyer who claimed that morals were only for the "middle class females". He claimed that the poor could not afford morals and ethics, and the wealthy didn't have to abide by them. He claimed that he had read am article that claimed

2

that about 40% of men were psychopaths and sociopaths. I remember teasing him and asking him which category he belonged to.

It was an eye opener for me. I have engaged many people in discussions concerning morals and ethics since that time. Think about it: If you were a mother who couldn't afford to feed your children – what morals would you be willing to override in order to get food for your starving children?

On the other hand, think about how many actors/musicians/ politicians/CEOs you have heard about, that committed crimes and didn't have to 'pay their debts to society' or simply "got their hands slapped"? I don't know about you, but this really p*ss*s me off. Why are we all not held by the same law and the same level of accountability and responsibility?

Taking this issue even further, this same lawyer told me that morals, honor and integrity are upheld by middle class women. That doesn't say much for us men. When I questioned the lawyer about why he thought women tended to be more moral and honorable than men, he simply asked me: "How many men do you know who have had affairs? How many women do you know have had affairs? Why do you think there is such a difference between the genders?"

Apparently, the large difference between men engaging in affairs versus women engaging in affairs has dramatically decreased over the last couple of decades –

and that of course is interesting in and of itself. Why is it, that now that women have more education and more independence, they are engaging in more affairs? Is it because they are not afraid of being abandoned by their partners? They have more education and better paying jobs and can take of themselves?

Is it because they are no longer willing to take the "crap" that some men are known to dish to out, like addiction, alcoholism, abuse, affairs, etc.? Is it because they are waiting longer to have children or choosing not to have children at all? If they don't have children, they have less of a worry about their husbands abandoning them and not having the means to take care of the children. Obviously if they chose not to have children, they only have to take care of themselves and the additional responsibilities are not there.

This lawyer also said, "Further, not all women abide by the same code of ethics or morality; some men are far more protective of their women and children than others; the majority of women have a huge "mother bear" attitude when it comes to protecting their children, others don't."

Much later in my life, I brought up the issue of morality and men (I didn't ask about women) to one of the practitioners at the Gibson clinic (I will explain later). He explained how many more men are sociopaths and psychopaths when compared to women. Hmmm, interesting. I wonder why?

But I am getting off the track here – let's go back to how there are people with money and in a position of power who are willing to take advantage of the average Joe with misleading or false information. This is my big issue right now. Why? Because I was misled by my physician who was mislead by Big Pharma. AND, I paid the price. I paid the price not just from my wallet but also with my health.

Like most people I was brought up to believe that physicians were well trained and had my best interests at heart. While some may have my best interests at heart, we are finding out that many of them don't. Further, they are not well trained at all. In fact, for the most part Big Pharma is in control of their training and Big Pharma definitely does not have my optimal health as their bottom line. In fact, if they did have my optimal health as their underlying concern, they might be out of business!!

If, on the other hand, they teach MDs to put me on drugs for the rest of my life; drugs that will probably deplete my body of nutrients; drugs that they actually know will lead to further prescriptions; then I keep paying them and they stay in business.

Did you know that Big Pharma has no legal responsibility for your health but does have a legal responsibility to make their shareholders money? That in and of itself says a lot.

So here I was at 68 years of age. I was diagnosed with Alzheimer's and put on drugs that would "help prevent the disease from getting worse". Note that the drugs were not meant to solve the problem but rather keep it from getting worse. But even that didn't happen – it did get worse. If I had continued on the path my MD had started me on, I would still be on lots of different pharmaceutical medications. The drugs would continue to cause more issues. The additional symptoms provoking the MD to prescribe more prescriptions to manage the additional symptoms, again symptoms the drugs themselves created. And of course, I would have been paying for all the prescriptions for the rest of my life.

WOW! I am so glad that I chose to alter the pathway and create a different life experience.

Prescriptions to manage symptoms isn't the only issue here. Another huge factor involved in this process is that Alzheimer's is hugely misdiagnosed!! At one point, I started to laugh, if I added up all the types of misdiagnoses and count up all the percentages of misdiagnoses – there isn't any room left for Alzheimer's! Not only are there other types of dementia –there are over 100 different types of dementia currently being researched. Different causes, different protocols, different results. They all require different treatment protocols. In addition, there are all kinds of causes of dementia – many of which can be easily resolved!!! And without prescription drugs.

But here I was. Sitting on couch. Fading away. Wasting my retirement funds on prescription drugs. Supporting Big Pharma. Again, at cost to both my pocket book and my health!!

So, what happened to me? My daughter and son-in-law have a great relationship with a clinic of practitioners who work with REAL medicine rather than synthetic artificial medication, i.e. prescriptions. REAL medicine gave me my health back.

The Clinic is run by the Gibson family. Each practitioner in the family has a different set of degrees and/or designations in the healing arts. They are dedicated to learning, exploring and applying REAL medicine to their clients. They work as a team keeping each other up to date on all the really "good" science out there.

They pride themselves on always keeping up with and/or ahead of the latest "good" research. They do not get carried away with trends that have little impact; and they understand research design and analysis. Consequently, they are in a position to look at a given study and determine whether it was an appropriate design, whether the proper analysis was applied, whether they had a sufficient sample sizes, whether the researchers were claiming relative risk verses absolute risk, whether it was a correlation or a causal process, and lots of other factors. Of course, as we have all come to know, one variable that has a huge impact is who is funding the research? AND, who is paying to get the research published?

That is why I keep saying "good" research. Way too much of current medical research is really poor research. As you will find throughout this book, even top people in "Conventional" Medicine are now recognizing that much of the research is ineffective research.

But it goes further than the research. As a result of poor research, clinic practices and protocols in Western medicine are ineffective. Even worse, many of the clinic protocols have never even been clinically studied!! They don't even know the mechanism of action of most of prescription drugs – it is hypothesized, suggested or indicated but actually unknown!!

What we do hear is that Western medicine is "evidenced based" medicine. When you hear, "evidenced based" medicine – what does that mean for you?

It certainly carried a huge level of weightedness for me. When I say weight, I mean authority, importance, and significance.

We also think that when clinical studies or articles are "peer reviewed" that also means that they carry a lot of weight. That other researchers in the area have reviewed them and accept them as having quality and application. I certainly thought that.

The problem is, I keep learning that this "evidence based" medicine is far too often NOT "evidenced based" and that peer reviewed simply means it was sent to peers who they know will agree with them. And far too often, that is corrupted by the almighty dollar. What a lot of hogwash!!!

What I am finding out is nothing short of amazing. One of the things that 'really blew my mind' so to speak, was that the Editor in Chiefs of two of the most prestigious medical journals were claiming 50% of medical research was out right wrong and the other 50% was questionable. And we are taught to trust the Western Medical Profession? That alone really made me angry and also pushed me to get to the bottom of things.

The prestigious medical journals I am talking about are the **Lancet** and **the New England Journal of Medicine.** Any article or study that gets published in them has to make its way past the Editor in Chief. It is a natural assumption for physicians to make, never mind us lay people, that if clinical trials and studies get into journals like these, they must have a lot of credence behind them. Right?? Wrong!!

I am going to share with you what the Editor in Chiefs of both the *Lancet* and the *New England Journal of Medicine* wrote. This will set the framework for this book. From there, I will go into all kinds of medical arenas and reveal things every physician and lay person SHOULD know, but don't.

Dr. Richard Horton, Editor-in-Chief of the **Lancet**, one of the most prestigious medical journals in the world, stated:

> The case against science is straightforward: much of the scientific literature, perhaps half, may simply be untrue. Afflicted by studies with small sample sizes, tiny effects, invalid exploratory analyses, and flagrant conflicts of interest, together with an obsession for pursuing fashionable trends of dubious importance, science has taken a turn towards darkness.[1]

If that wasn't bad enough, the Editor in Chief of the **New England Journal of Medicine**, Dr. Marcia Angell, said virtually the same thing:

> The problems I've discussed are not limited to psychiatry, although they reach their most florid form there. Similar conflicts of interest and biases exist in virtually every field of medicine, particularly those that rely heavily on drugs or devices. It is simply no longer possible to believe much of the clinical research that is published, or to rely on the judgment of trusted physicians or authoritative medical guidelines. I take no pleasure in this conclusion, which I reached slowly and reluctantly

over my two decades as an editor of The New England Journal of Medicine.[2]

Another hugely powerful statement written in the same article,

> Many drugs that are assumed to be effective *are probably little better than placebos*, but there is no way to know because negative results are hidden. …reviews of every placebo-controlled clinical trial submitted for initial approval of the six most widely used antidepressant drugs approved between 1987 and 1999 – Prozac, Paxil, Zoloft, Celexa, Serzone, and Effexor. They found that on average, placebos were 80% as effective as the drugs. The difference between drug and placebo was so small that it was unlikely to be of any clinical significance.[3]

I should clarify here the above quote was made with regards to psychiatry and predominantly anti-depressants, however, it is becoming apparent that the same issues apply across all fields of medicine. Dr. Marcia Angell published a very revealing book, *The Truth About Drug Companies: How They Deceive Us and What to Do About It.*

Wow! I couldn't believe it. How far do the cover ups go? How wide did they extend? I needed to know the answers to these questions. But what resources could I trust? Where could I start to look? My mind was reeling with questions.

I continued to read the articles. The more I read, the more I realized there were all kinds of reasons the research could not be trusted.

I had a lot of research I needed to do. I started with a self-reflection of my own journey. Years of wasting away in front of a television, spending money on drugs that were obviously not resolving the problem. MDs telling me it was part of aging and there was nothing I could do about it.

Yet, when I went on a particular healthy diet that specified certain combinations of foods at certain times, eliminate some toxic metals from my body, and take a few supplements and within months I was back up and functioning again! I got my brain back! I was no longer fading away in front of the television. I regained my cognitive clarity, memory, and energy. What a difference. That is huge!!

Consequently, I am up and fully functioning again. I am no longer supporting Big Pharma at cost to my body. Rather I am now engaged in unraveling all the unethical, immoral, irresponsibilities of our medical system and in particular of Big Pharma.

This is a big break for me. As I already explained, my passion is researching underlying political and financial maneuvers, I am investigating and researching again. This time, however, I am applying my passion to uncovering Big Pharma's underlying agendas.

So, I wait patiently, on the phone. On the other end is a university professor who promised to give me some leads, anonymously. It took me forever to connect with him, so I didn't want to take the risk of waiting for him to call me back. A student interrupted our call and I told him I would wait no matter how long it took.

As much as I love doing the research, I love feeling like my old self again. Unfortunately, I don't love what I am finding. What I am researching is making me angry and truly 'pi*s*d off' to put it nicely.

My research isn't just about my journey into and out of disease. It is also my father's journey.

My father died of cancer when I was a young man in my twenties. It was a tormented time of watching the man I looked up to and admired both as a child and as a young man, die a long, drawn-out, and agonizing death. He was in and out of chemotherapy; looking more and more frail. Losing his hair was the easy part; the agonizing pain, the most difficult part. Never mind the nausea and vomiting and other symptoms in between. I couldn't do anything to help except sit by him and watch the invisible monster slowly kill my father and best friend.

With the research I am now engaged in, I am finding that they are now understanding that cancer is actually a wide variety of diseases that have been collected under the "cancer" umbrella term. That not only are there different cancers in different areas of the body,

13

but there are even many different types of cancers/disorders within a given area of the body. Consequently, there are many different protocols that can work. There is one book out there that identifies over 100 different protocols for different types of cancers, and they are all based on healthy options rather than chemotherapy and radiation. Wow!!

Now I learn that there are all kinds of treatment protocols that could have helped my father. But like most of us, I trusted the Western medical sciences. It never occurred to me, back then, how backwards and how misinformed oncologists, never mind all the other types of MDs, were as a profession. Or how long it takes for good science to actually reach the physicians and be applied in hospitals.

I didn't suffer the physically agonizing death my father suffered. I suffered on an entirely different level. But both my father and I waited for death to happen rather than living life to its fullest. He died a slow death physically while I died a slow death mentally.

Both of us had entrusted our lives to physicians who didn't know how to resolve the problem because they were only trained to prescribe synthetic artificial compounds that, as it turns out, are detrimental to the body.

I always believed my MD was a well-trained professional in the field. I believed I could trust him and depend on his knowledge and his expertise.

Obviously, I was wrong. Who could I trust? Where should I start? What about the Gibson Clinic? They were the ones who got me off all the drugs. They didn't want to take my money for the rest of my life to *'manage my symptoms'*. Instead, they *'eliminated the underlying problem'*.

Naturally, I made an appointment with the Gibson Clinic. When I met with the practitioners at the Clinic, I asked where I should start my research and investigation. They laughed and suggested I start by looking at how the body functions. That didn't make sense to me, but I followed their direction.

It has been estimated that we:

- Make over two billion red blood cells every minute
- Make over a litre of saliva daily
- Make 3 to 4 quarts of hydrochloric acid daily
- Make 0.5 litres of cerebral spinal fluid daily

And that we keep renewing:

- About 50 million white blood cells to protect us
- Over 100 types of neurotransmitters
- Over 75,000 enzymes
- Our skin every 6 months
- Our liver every 6 weeks

Our stomach lining every 4 days and the aspect of the stomach that is in contact with our food, every 5 minutes

We also keep replacing:

- Our nails about 6 months
- Eye lashes every 150 days
- Compounds like CoQ10 & glutathione constantly

There are different types of glutathione compounds and they are involved in a huge number of functions throughout the body and have to be made inside of every cell. And these lists went on and on.

If the body has to do all of that and so much more, then we need to ask, what does the body require to keep up all that phenomenal work? What materials does the body require to make all of these compounds and fluids? Food material, obviously; and in food, we find the following raw materials:

- Alkaloids: indoles, isoquinolines, piperdines, purines, quinolizidines, tropanes
- Amino acids (22 amino acids)
- Anti-oxidants (glutathiones, SOD, carotenoids, flavonoids, allylsulfides, polyphenols, etc.)
- Carotenoids
- Essential fatty acids
- Fats/lipids/waxes/sterols/monoglycerids/diglyceri des/triglerides/phospholipids, etc.
- Fiber: soluble, non-soluble glycosides

- Minerals: calcium, chloride, magnesium, phosphorus, potassium, sodium, sulfur
- Phenolics: polyphenols, coumarins, flavonoids, lignans, phenolics, quinones, stilbenes, tannins
- Sugars: fructose, glucose, sucrose, etc.
- Sulfides
- Terpenes: diterpenes, iridoid, monoterpenes, sesquesterpenes, triterpenes
- Trace minerals: chromium, copper, fluoride, iodine, iron, manganese, molybdenum, selenium, zinc
- Vitamins: A, Bs, C, D, E, Ks

To name a few.

If the body isn't functioning effectively, it is probably either lacking a given compound (nutrient(s)) from food to do the job, OR it needs to get rid of something (toxin(s)) preventing the body from achieving what it needs to achieve. That sounds pretty logical and straight forward. Actually, it goes right back to the father of Western Medicine, Hippocrates who said, *'Food is your medicine and medicine is your food.'*

Whether you believe in some Creationism theory or some Evolution theory or some combination...our bodies were designed to work in cooperation with nature. Nature feeds us, supports us, nurtures us, and heals us. Our body's enzymes and cellular receptors were designed to work in accordance with compounds found in nature. It makes sense regardless of your spiritual/non-spiritual beliefs.

So how did we get from using "REAL" medicine to deal with illness, to artificial synthetic compounds (Big Pharma) the body isn't designed to work with?

Easy, follow the money. Of course, there is a lot more involved than just greed; there is power, control, government officials, underhanded processes, illegal activities, marketing, miscommunication and a whole lot more.

My first question was, "Well surely MDs are taught about food, herbs and spices and all the nutrition our bodies require?" Would you believe they are not?!!?!!

That is where my research started: Why they are *not* taught about the nutrient requirements the body requires? Why they are *not* taught about all the toxins in our food, in the soils, and in the air we breathe or the water we drink?

That is where this all gets interesting, especially for an old man like me who was bought up to believe in the system and that all the Complementary and Alternative was non-evidenced flaky stuff? Now I look back and question myself, "What the heck was I thinking?"

Well the answer is simple. I wasn't thinking. I made a very inaccurate assumption. I assumed MDs were taught all this basic, logical stuff! They are not. The first failing, if you will, of our medical system.

Before I started the next step of my investigation I had to sit down and figure out the questions I wanted answered first.

- What are our medical professionals taught?
- Who determines what they are taught?
- Who determines their protocol and procedure?
- Who does the research?
- How long does it take for the research to make it to the MDs and/or university curriculums and/or hospitals?
- What gets into the medical journals and who decides and based on what variables?

I had to keep looking. Surely it wasn't all that bad. Then I read what Dr. Robert Horton, of the *New England Journal of Medicine* who stated:

> The apparent endemicity of bad research behaviour is alarming. In their quest for telling a compelling story, scientists too often sculpt data to fit their preferred theory of the world. Or they retrofit hypotheses to fit their data. Journal editors deserve their fair share of criticism too.[4]

Okay, so these are pretty powerful statements. And they are made by people in powerful positions who should know. I needed to find someone who actually did the research to back up these kinds of statements. Dr Jane from the Gibsons Clinic told me to look into Dr. Ioannidis' research saying that he is well known in the medical field. He has an impressive background, he

19

is a Stanford professor considered to be, "one of the most influential scientists alive...For the last 20 years, he has amazed an internationally regarded body of research about all the ways science isn't actually science-based."[5]

Dr. Ioannidis analyzed 49 studies and wrote the following:

> 49 of the most highly regarded research findings in medicine over the previous 13 years, as judged by the science community's two standard measures: the papers had appeared in the journals most widely cited in research articles, and the 49 articles themselves were the most widely cited articles in these journals," he found that "between a third and a half of the most acclaimed research in medicine was proven untrustworthy...[6,7]

I couldn't believe it. Over a third of the most acclaimed research was proven wrong!?

Now I needed to find out who I could trust. And so, began the investigation. I focused on what the Ancient Greek literature taught, 'you need to pursue truth, no matter what that truth might be'.

Chapter 2
The Internet?

I know there is a lot of misleading information on the internet, but I thought I would start there first anyway, and it was quite interesting. I had no idea how many conflicting pieces of information are on the internet. So, I started another list of questions:

- How much is nonsense?

- How much is regurgitated crap?

- How does one sort the weeds from the plants of value?

One thing I found that really angered me is that research is biased towards those who fund the study. Many of us would like to believe if we are dealing with scientists, professional people who are trained to be objective, then we are dealing with people who are moral and ethical. That is not necessarily the case.

The old saying, "Follow the money", is more apparent than ever. It is not necessarily that the scientists are immoral creatures, rather scientists are responsible to a university or a corporation. If that institution or organization is dependent on, or subsidized by, research grants, then there is going to be pressure to provide the results requested.

In addition, if a given scientist or professor is looking to make a name or get a series of publications for his CV (a CV is the professional name for a resume, it includes publications and other components a regular resume does not have) in order to get tenure, he is going to do what he needs to do to achieve that.

Remember, he probably has a mortgage to pay, student loans to repay, a family to support, and bills to pay, just the like the rest of us. If he doesn't cooperate and do what he is told to do, he may not be able to make his personal responsibilities. Does that make him a bad guy? Where do morals and ethics fit in? You have to determine that for yourself.

When I talked with Dr. Jane about it, she told me of a couple of situations she had been in where she was told to alter the findings of her study to meet the requirements of an Executive Director for whom she was doing the paper. She refused to make the unethical adjustments and her contract was not renewed a couple of months later.

Morals; honor; integrity; where is the line? I kept looking.

I found an article on newscientist.com in which study leader Joel Lexchin told New Scientist:

Researchers analysed 30 previous reports examining pharmaceutical industry-backed research and found the conclusions of such research were four times more likely to be positive than research backed by other sponsors. What we found was that in almost all cases there was a bias, a rather heavy bias, in favour [of a drug] when the study was industry funded.[8]

Dr. Horton basically said the same thing:

Universities are in a perpetual struggle for money and talent, endpoints that foster reductive metrics, such as high-impact publication. National assessment procedures, such as the Research Excellence Framework, incentivise bad practices.[9]

Dr. John Ioannidis, a Stanford University Professor, spoke in front of Harvard University MDs and said, "In science, we are very eager to make big stories, big claims," he opened his lecture, with a mischievous grin, "the question is: are those claims accurate?" According to Ioannidis, the answer, "at least most of the time, is an unequivocal 'no.'"[10]

Dr. Ioannidis charges that,

...as much as 90 percent of the published medical information that doctors rely on is flawed. His work has been widely accepted by the medical community; it has been published in the field's top journals, where it is heavily cited; and he is a big draw at conferences.[11]

According to the *The Guardian*:

> The study, **Published on Monday in the Proceedings of the National Academy of Sciences** (PNAS), found that more than two-thirds of the biomedical and life sciences papers that have been retracted from the scientific record are due to misconduct by researchers, rather than error.

> The results add weight to **recent concerns that scientific misconduct is on the rise** and that fraud increasingly affects fields that underpin many areas of public concern, such as medicine and healthcare.[12]

Finding that misconduct and fraud are on the rise certainly wasn't encouraging.

I thought maybe if I went into a given field of medicine, I might find a different perspective. I looked for a commentary on cancer. I found Dr. Morten Oksvold of the University of Oslo, who explored false data in cancer research and found that one quarter of research papers, contained false data.[13]

Okay, so what if I looked at institutions rather than fields of medicine? I found a Charles Piller, who wrote an article on Statnews.com claiming Stanford

University and other prestigious medical research institutions have "flagrantly violated a federal law requiring public reporting of study results," and "the worst offenders included four of the top 10 recipients of federal medical research funding from the National Institutes of Health: Stanford, the University of Pennsylvania, the University of Pittsburgh, and the University of California, San Diego. All disclosed research results late, or not at all, at least 95 percent of the time since reporting became mandatory in 2008."[14]

Once again that wasn't encouraging. So rather than look at a field of medicine, or an institution, how about if I looked at the individual physicians? I came across a Dr. Athinia Tatsioni, University of Ioannina, who claimed, "usually what happens is that the doctor will ask for a suite of biochemical tests—liver fat, pancreas function, and so on... The tests could turn up something, but they're probably irrelevant. Just having a good talk with the patient and getting a close history is much more likely to tell me what's wrong."[15]

I then found a PowerPoint presentation produced by Dr. Ted Colton, Professor & Chair Emeritus, and Department of Epidemiology & Biostatistics, which elaborated even more on the fraud in Medical Research.[16]

"Shoot!" I thought to myself. So how do we figure out what and who we can trust and what is questionable? Most of us do not have PhDs in Research, Design and

Analysis, so my next stop was going back to Dr. Jane. She does have a PhD in Research Design and Analysis and her first doctorate thesis was entitled: *Psycho neuroendocrinology*. Maybe she could help clarify the questions we need to ask. She would probably be able to direct me to good research sources. She might even be able to provide some of the answers.

Chapter 3

More research issues than meets the eye

Personally, I figured the problems in research simply had to do with "follow the money". The research would be biased to whoever was providing the funds to the research. As unfortunate as that is, we know scientists are people who want to keep their jobs. When working for universities, their position depends on the amount of funding they bring in. The same pressure is also found in other institutions and corporations.

Obviously, we all have to pay our bills, but at what price? We used to laugh at lawyers 'selling their souls' to the big legal companies. It sounds like the scientists are 'selling their souls' as well.

When I dug a little deeper, I found research claiming that even with scientists who do have moral and ethical virtues, they will unwittingly, or unconsciously, support the funder. There are a number of sites discussing how the grant agencies actually end up reinforcing this paradigm.

In the UK, the government launched a review to improve university research funding. Lord Stern, the president of the British Academy, stated "Research assessment should not unwittingly introduce incentives for perverse behaviour, nor should it be overly burdensome."[17]

Okay, so pressure to get funding for research and from peer pressure can impact on a scientist consciously and unconsciously. Scientists are not as objective as we would like them to be. That really sucks when you go to a physician who wants to put you on a medication. Is it really going to do what it is acclaimed to do, or are you going to simply be supporting Big Pharma?

As I worked through my investigation, I came to understand a lot more about research, design and analysis, never mind marketing, than I had ever wanted to. Yet, on the other hand, it gave me a much better understanding of many issues that can go sideways or be manipulated in the process of researching a compound, getting it formulated and then to the marketplace. Scientists have an incredible amount of leeway they can play with. It is really scary.

In this chapter, I am going to give you a little bit of my understanding of the actual research issues being played with. In the next chapter, I am going to provide you with just a glimpse of how marketing can manipulate, not only the lay person, but also the physicians!

In subsequent chapters, I am going to deal with research issues in specific areas of medicine.

Let's start out with the obvious: drug companies have to put out a lot of money to support research. Research, in and of itself, is expensive. We all get that.

Consequently, there are shortcuts and a lot of the shortcuts cause misleading results.

I obviously don't have a degree in research, design and analysis. What I did was take the information I could gain from the internet and summarize it myself. Then I ran it by Dr. Daniel from the Gibson Clinic, who has a PhD in Nutrition, to correct any misconceptions.

Finally, I ran it by my wife, Mary, to see if she could understand what I was saying. Now I am providing it in these very simple terms so you can understand them. I will review the steps to designing a research study and give you an idea of many issues that exist and the types of analyses that can be used. Remember, at each step of the way, data can be manipulated.

Hypothesis
A study begins with the hypothesis. A statement that needs to be confirmed or denied. Unfortunately, too many studies have a problem with this very first step.

For instance, your study might be whether or not a given drug reduces cholesterol. However, when the basic premise is that cholesterol is bad and therefore needs to be reduced, with no research to see if cholesterol is good, then whether the drug does what it is acclaimed to do is irrelevant. In fact, the most recent research reveals how the whole cholesterol issue is irrelevant, clearly illustrating a "Cholesterol Myth."

For instance, there are all kinds of HDL and even more types of LDL. It is a lot more complex than physicians were led to believe. The point, however, is that the hypothesis was based on an incorrect assumption.

Going back to the above assumption leads to a very basic question, "how is the "bad cholesterol" research of any value?" It isn't. The body needs all kinds of cholesterols and the liver oversees that. For good reason.

Another issue fitting in with the Cholesterol Myth is whether fats are good or bad for you. The assumption that was taught, was all fats are bad for you because they cause weight gain and cardio issues. Well, this whole arena concerning fats has been turned around and dumped on its head. There are good fats and bad fats. Further, what was once thought to be a bad fat is now considered to be a good fat. Why are there so many contradictions? Let's move on.

When we were taught that all fats were bad and caused weight gain, without realizing that the body needed good healthy fats, which also break down fats, we started eating fat free food. Oh crap. These fat free foods cause even more problems!! You see, to make the fat free food taste good they replaced the fat with sugars and synthetic compounds, some of which are toxic to the body. Which of course stimulates the release of insulate, provokes storage of fats, and encourages inflammation throughout the body. So, these fat free foods actually cause obesity and diabetes!! Never mind the additional chemical flavourings and preservatives.

In addition, they actually rob the body of nutrients. Yeah, that's right! Those toxins actually block your body from absorbing the nutrients you need.

There is also the issue that healthy fats do make you feel full. When you don't consume healthy fats and consume even more sugar and other toxins, you are left feeling hungry and consequently eat more but absorb less thanks to the toxins.

It is amazing how we have been conned. And we fell for it, because we didn't know any better. Actually, neither did most of the physicians!

Another good example are anti-depressants. They are based on the hypothesis that low serotonin (a neurotransmitter) levels cause depression. Therefore, regulating serotonin would eliminate depression, right? Well, the real research shows:

- Low serotonin levels have never been shown to cause depression;
- Regulating serotonin levels with drugs has never been shown to eliminate depression;

- Most anti-depressants are no more effective than a placebo; and
- Some anti-depressants are known to provoke suicidal ideation and behavior.

Hey, I thought physicians prescribed anti-depressants for depression? Oh crap, again.

Not only that, but I found all kinds of research showing that there are all kinds of nutrient deficiencies, gut issues, and various toxins (insecticides pesticides herbicides, POPs (persistent organic pollutants), heavy metals, etc.) that are well recognized for causing depression! Shouldn't a good physician be looking at addressing all these other issues rather than simply prescribing an anti-depressant that ends up masking the underlying problem?

Yes, these and many other issues are prevalent with anti-depressant drugs and research. But, perhaps one of the biggest issues is that any given anti-depressant drug makes over a million dollars a day!! When you are in the money-making business, why would you want to inform your key marketers, i.e., the physicians, of what is really going on?

Remember that Dr. Richard Norton of the **Lancet** said, "Afflicted by studies with small sample sizes, tiny effects, invalid exploratory analyses, and flagrant conflicts of interest, together with an **obsession for pursuing fashionable trends** of dubious importance, science has taken a turn towards darkness."[18]

Yup, I guess that fits in here, don't you think? And I blindly believed in all of this medical stuff? Nuts! But let's keep going, I haven't finished here yet.

Design

The next part of an investigation is determining what kind of design one should use. I am not going to go into all the issues playing into what determines the most effective design of study. It looks like that could take a full book in, and of, itself. I am going to scan over the basic kinds of designs and make a generalized statement: unfortunately, too often the wrong kind of design is utilized.

Some designs are very costly and others, obviously, substantially less. In theory, funding should not get in the way of the appropriate design for a medical formula, but it does:

- Double blind (meaning no one knows what the study is about)
- Cross over (the participants were tracked when they both used the given drug and then when they didn't)
- Double blind, cross over study: Considered the golden study
- Randomized controlled trials: the most commonly used
- Case study: a single subject study

- Was there a control group - if so, what variables were controlled for?
- Was there a control group, or was the drug compared to another drug or perhaps both?
- Controlled observational studies
- Uncontrolled observational studies
- Longitudinal studies
- Systematic reviews
- Meta-analysis

Historically, most agreed the double blind and cross over studies were the golden measure in medical research. Today, however, researchers like Dr. Ioannidis have established concerns even with the double-blind cross over study:

- Far too often, far too few subjects are utilized to make any kind of conclusion
- Lack of demographic controls (cigarette smoking, alcohol consumption, caffeine intake, etc.)
- Food and drug interactions are rarely taken into consideration
- Toxicity levels already in the body
- Recruitment of subjects can produce distorted population biases
- Lingering effects in the cross over studies may impact the results
- Withdrawal effects may produce confounding variables

- Some drugs may not be conducive to cross over research designs

Hopefully I haven't bored you to tears yet. I hope you got as interested in all of this stuff, like I did. It makes you wonder, well, let's say it made me wonder, about all the different drugs on the market.

- Were they researched properly? Meaning, did they have a meaningful hypothesis, proper design & analysis, etc.
- How do know who and what to trust? Do they do what Pharma claims they do, and are they safe?
- How do we help the physician and the general public be aware of these issues? I am certainly doing my best!

Dr Jane shared that one of her professors told her that any good researcher knows how to get positive results with poorly designed studies. That's scary.

Let's keep going, there are a few other issues to take into consideration, like how the information is collected.

Laboratory testing

Although considered objective testing there are a number of tests that are considered useless, for example:

- If blood tests are so accurate, then why is the FDA now giving the PSA a "D" rating because the false negatives (saying everything is good when it isn't) and false positives (saying there is an issue when there isn't) are over 80%.

- The CA-125 blood test that is used to detect ovarian cancer in women has a high level of inaccuracy.
- Dr. Carolyn Dean claims a Magnesium test is completely useless.
- Another test deemed useless is for Vitamin B12 levels.
- While a calcium blood test may be accurate, it is more indicative of a metabolic disorder than insufficient calcium.
- Thyroid tests may show up abnormal, but it is usually a problem with the adrenals and/or the liver.
- Apart from blood analysis, what about the fact a mammogram can't tell the difference between a fat cell and a cancer cell and consequently the FDA has also given mammograms a 'D' rating.

Questionnaires

They are obviously more subjective and have a number of issues that need to be considered:

- Were the questions open ended or closed?

- Were the questionnaires piloted – which is like a pretesting to determine if the questions gave the information required?
- Were the questions designed to reflect the current situation or a lifelong situation?
- Were the interviewers properly trained?
- What about the timing of the study, i.e., if seasonal issues like hay fever or SADs are accounted for?

Stress levels

What about the stress level of the participant before, during and after the study? Even the stress of going to see an MD can increase blood pressure tests and consequently is called the "White Coat Affect".

Today, apparently your hand grip provides more information than your blood pressure when it comes to predicting mortality and morbidity.

The time of day

Our bodies work on 24-hour rhythms – called circadian rhythms, and the time of day can alter a number of testing procedures (blood tests, blood pressure, blood glucose levels, etc.).

- Were all the subjects tested at the same time of day?
- Was each individual subject tested at the same time each day?
- Exercise can affect many physiological variables. What physical activity does the client normally

participate in? Whether or not they had come from the gym.

- The types of food a person eats can cause drugs to break down faster or prevent them from breaking down.
- If clients dropped out of the study, we need to know why.

Number of subjects

Of course, there is the concern about how many participants there were.

- A case study is based on one participant.
- A group study may have anywhere between 2 and hundreds of thousands.

There are a huge number of articles on the internet and from medical journals claiming the number of subjects is far too small to make the conclusions they are making.

On the other hand, there are various studies that have a huge number of people but too few controls in the study to make it of value.

Both the issue being investigated, and the design of the study need to be taken into consideration to determine how many subjects need to be in the study in order to make valid conclusions. Repeatedly I have read, too many conclusions are based on an inadequate number of participants in the study.

Duration

I have to tell you, I had fun thinking about this issue. Duration can be thought of from various different perspectives.

The first is the duration of the study. When we are dealing with a given design for a new drug, how long is a drug tested for? Longer test durations are more helpful in determining side affects but are costlier. Or how long is a given drug required to be tested before it is approved? It comes down to money, again. If cutting costs is important to the researcher, the study will be shorter.

This is important because the studies typically determine how long you need to be on the medication to eliminate a symptom.

When I started to read about the different issues resulting from having too short or too long a time period, I started to laugh. It is one thing for a physician to tell you to take an anti-biotic for two weeks. It is another thing entirely when people simply accept that they are going to be on a medication for life. This applies to blood pressure medication, a statin, an anti-inflammatory, a hypothyroid, an anti-diabetic, or whatever other pharmaceutical.

Another question to ask is do the studies ever determine when you can get off the medication? Remember they make a lot of money just managing symptoms rather than eliminating the cause!! They don't really have motivation to study what happens when the medication is stopped.

It's interesting how much we just don't even bother to think through. We have a problem; we go to an MD; he asks a couple of questions; he gives us a prescription; we take it. I hate to have to admit I just never thought about what went into the research and design. I had no idea there were so many issues. I didn't question my physician's training in research, design and analysis, nor did I question the Big Pharma, or how and why a given physician may prescribe a given drug.

Now I am questioning everything. AND, I am questioning myself and how I could have been so blindly accepting.

Remember they make a lot of money just managing symptoms rather than eliminating the cause!!

Uncontrolled variables

What about the health concerns of the participants prior to the study?

- For instance, in some of the anti-depressant trials the participants were healthy college students. How does one determine the benefit of an anti-depressant when it is prescribed for a healthy person?
- What if the subject has a number of health issues that could confound the results?
- What if the subject is also seeing a Dr. of Natural Medicine, Herbalist, Acupuncturist, Ayurveda practitioner, Naturopath, Nutritionist, etc.
- What consideration is given to drug and drug/or natural medicine interactions?

Dr Jane said she has seen many clients who were having problems because the drugs they were prescribed were interacting and causing even more problems! Prescriptions can also interact with natural remedies and diet, i.e. grapefruit.

Inappropriate data collection

In reviewing the manner in which the drug was researched, this one really threw me for a loop. Here are a couple of the more obvious examples of inappropriate data collection.

Research on birth control pills initially used rats and rabbits, neither of which have menstrual cycles. Then researchers for pharmaceutical companies used women in Puerto Rico as guinea pigs. It was marketed as safe, despite no prior research identifying any risk factors. In fact, many of the women did not even know they were taking part in a trial study. Tragically, three women died during from it during the first phase of the study.

A second example is the use of horse urine to create the medication used in Hormone Replacement Therapy is laughable. Humans are unable to absorb a horse estrogen. So, the data they collected was meaningless.

This is just nuts!!!

Statistical Analysis

Once we determine whether it is an appropriate research design, then we ask whether the analysis was appropriate. I started to research this part and decided I needed more help. I talked with Dr. Jim and Dr. Jane, from the Gibson Clinic. A couple of their statements stand out for me.

1. One study cannot prove everything.

Okay, that makes sense. There are simply too many confounding issues to look at even with just one drug and replication is important.

2. The *second* issue is complex and provoked a few more profound questions.
   a. Are there any assumptions in the initial hypothesis that need to be resolved first?
   b. Is the study proving what they claim it is proving?
   c. Are the design and the analysis the appropriate?

And further how do these issues impact on:

d. The FDA
e. What they tell physicians
f. The patient

But let's get back to the actual analysis. As the old saying goes, 'figures don't lie until statisticians start to figure'. There are a variety of different types of analysis that can be used in research. The two main types commonly used are correlational and MANOVAs. The most useful, a canonical, isn't used.

I'm not a statistician so let's just do a brief overview to get the gist of what is going on. If we understand the basic differences between these analysis types, then we can understand why the analysis can be so misleading.

Correlational research determines if there is a positive or negative correlation/relationship between two variables. Sounds logical, if I take the drug, the symptom disappears. However, the Gibsons would be more interested in finding out whether the cause of the symptom disappeared or simply the symptom was masked. The problem with correlational analysis is that it can be very misleading. Let's look at a simple example.

There is a positive correlation between people getting up and the sun rising however that doesn't mean the sun is causing people to get up. The children getting up or crying, the alarm going off, the dogs needing to go out, wanting to watch a special golf tournament on TV, needing to go to the bathroom, or a huge number of other variables may be responsible for people actually getting up. There is a positive **correlation** with the sun coming up as well, even though the sun didn't **cause** you to get up.

Unfortunately, many studies claim there is a causal relationship when there is only a correlational relationship. So, we need to be very careful about the kind of analysis used and the conclusions made.

A second problem is that even when studying different variables and using a more **causal** style analysis, it may still be an inappropriate analysis. The first type of analysis is a MANOVA, which looks at the relationship between two or more variables. But an even better causal analysis is the Canonical Analysis which looks at several factors, each factor containing several variables. Dr. Jane and Dr. Jim think this style of research design and analysis should typically be used in medical research as it provides the ability to look at several relationships simultaneously. However, it is the most expensive, which is why it is not often used.

Some of the psychological research has used this canonical style of analysis, but psychological research is also fraught with all kinds of similar issues as medical research. The canonicals will look at several factors and each factor may have several variables. The Canonical Analysis is only recently getting into medical research.

The Gibsons' perspective is that the body has so many different interactive systems and each system contains so many different types of tissues, cells and compounds, it is rather inappropriate to simply assess two simple variables to the exclusion of all the others. Even the rise and fall of most compounds in the body is going to have a variety of effects throughout the body. Consequently, simple correlational kinds of research make a mockery of a lot of medical research.

Another similar issue is the fact that so many studies don't address "hard" outcomes but rather "soft" outcomes or variables. Hard variables might involve issues like survival versus death. Whereas soft variables might address "self-reported symptoms". Big Pharma criticizes REAL medicine for using too many soft variables, yet Big Pharma itself is riddled with soft variable analysis.

Along with hard versus soft variable analysis, and correlational versus MANOVA & Canonical Analysis, is the issue of whether it was the drug that actually caused the improvement.

A good example of this kind of issue arises with all the diets for weight loss. As Dr. Daniel from the Gibson Clinic would say, virtually any diet will work for some, some of the time. Why, because it is not usually how the diet is designed, but rather other components. For instance, when people go on diets:

- They eliminate the fast foods, the junk foods, the pasteurized foods, and the microwaved foods.

- They will typically focus on simple whole foods (and protein shakes) and a small dinner.
- These eliminate a lot of calories, in particular, all of the bad kind of calories, such as junk food, processed food, microwaved food, etc.
- They often engage in more physical activity.

Consequently, the weight loss is more due to what they have eliminated in terms of foods and what they have added in terms of exercise, as opposed to the actual diet itself.

This lack of recognition of the contributing factors is huge in medical research. When these kinds of variables are taken into consideration a given diet, or pharmaceutical, loses its significant results. These issues are not recognized in the news headlines!!

Question posed

Another challenge with research is not about the type of analysis that is utilized, but rather the type of question being posed. For instance, is the drug effective compared to something else? When working with comparative analysis, they will often use competitive drugs to establish a more effective result.

- They deliberately use a drug that is known not to be effective, or an inferior drug.
- They utilize smaller dosages of the competitive drug in the trials.

- In the case of comparing a drug with a REAL medicine (food or herb) they use:
  - A species known to have less nutrient density
  - For a duration of time known to be ineffective, i.e. it may take three weeks to get enough in the system to have an affect
  - In a dosage below what is known to work

In cases like these, the drug company funding the research is ahead of the game before the data is even collected. The conclusions make headlines; the research design and analysis don't!!

Another type of question is one that addresses a correlation between a symptom and the use of a drug to manage the symptom.

Another issue needing to be addressed in research is posing questions regarding 'selective hot topics'. This includes topics that are:

- "Hot" in research such as research based on the assumption that low levels of serotonin cause depression.
- Based on "false premises" and hypotheses. For instance, research based on the assumption that cholesterol is bad for you or that all plaque in the arteries is caused by cholesterol.

Equipment used
Other issues have to do with the equipment that is used. For instance, it is well known that mammograms,

47

colonoscopies and PSA tests are loaded with interpretive interpretive inaccuracies. Usually, the stats reveal the false negatives and false positives run around 80%. This is partly why the FDA has given them a "D" rating over the past several years, despite the fact they are still being advertised.

When it comes to the mammograms, it is difficult to differentiate between fat cells and cancer cells. Yet, they are still being pushed on women today. I'll get more into this in the chapter on cancer research.

Individual Differences

This particular issue is huge for me, an old man who suffered with dementia. We know we are not all the same, but medical research appears to treat us as if we are.

- How does our mindset impact how our body functions?
- How does the pH in the gut impact how the body functions?
- How does the microbiota impact how the body functions?
- How does the current genetic profile of the individual impact how the body functions?
- How does our particular diet impact how our body functions?

These and so many other questions have a huge impact on the results of any given study. But unfortunately, they are not taken into consideration. We apparently now know the microbiota profile in your body is probably not the same as in my body, your microbiota profile is unique to you like your fingerprint. Consequently, something that may work for you and may work against me. Researchers are starting to recognize that this can have a huge impact on how an individual's system interacts with a given drug. One size does not fit all.

Opposing findings

How do we account for all the opposing findings in research? Let's look at a few examples where research contradicts itself.

- How is it that cell phones do, and don't, cause brain cancer?
- Supplements (across the board) are supposed to help eliminate a, b, c, and don't.
- How can a given drug be good for the heart, but also cause congestive heart failure, anti-depressants cause depression, chemotherapy causes cancer, etc.
- Drugs promoted to manage (note that doesn't say cure, only manage) diabetes cause even worse problems that can be fatal.
- The drug proclaimed as the be all and end all, has umpteen class action law suits against it or was taken off the market.

Due to the individual differences and the huge variety of causes for a given symptom profile or diagnosis, both opposing findings may be correct. Consequently, hypotheses posed, research, design and analysis become even more important to understand when making conclusions that impact our health and well-being.

When I did research on the drugs that I was prescribed, I not only found that there was a good probability that I was misdiagnosed, but also the drugs prescribed were known to exacerbate the issues and make matters worse.

Subsequent findings

A whole other concern is about drugs that are passed by the FDA and then recalled after repeated tragic consequences. For example, it may take over 500 deaths before they consider recalling a drug.

Do you know that there are 3 categories of drug recalls?

Class 1 Recall: when there is a reasonable probability the use of a drug will cause serious adverse health consequences or death.

Class II Recall: when the use of a given drug may cause temporary or medically reversible health consequences, but the probability of serious adverse health consequences is remote.

Class III Recall: when the use of a given drug is not likely to cause adverse health consequences.

This one really got my attention. I wanted to know if I was taking a drug that had serious consequences. I found a chart on a website that provides the number and class of drug recalls by the FDA that you might want to take a look at.[19]

What I found particularly interesting was that in 2004, a total of 166 drugs were recalled. The number of recalled drugs steadily increases up to 2015 where the number of recalls hit a high of 2,028. Thankfully, the two subsequent years show decreasing numbers.[20]

I am sure you have the same question I had: if all these drugs are supposed to go through rigorous research and umpteen trials before being okayed by the FDA – how come so many are being recalled!!?? If you are questioning the drug you are taking, make sure you look for drug recalls on the internet.

Reporting

A major issue with medical research is the reporting process. Most studies showing negative results are not reported to the FDA, only the positive results. And, of course, your physician only hears the positive results. Who wants to publish negative results?

I found out that Big Pharma, scientists and researchers are required to pay to publish an article in a medical journal. Consequently, as much research now reveals, most research is not published due to failure to provide significant positive results. Unfortunately, this type of publication protocol reinforces the use of poor statistical research, design and analysis so that researchers and universities maintain their grant support from Big Pharma.

As I noted previously, research is costly. Now I find out that publication is costly as well.

Perhaps the even bigger consequence is that the FDA focuses on the positive published results to determine approval status. This, of course, means that Big Pharma profits at the cost of our health and our pocketbooks.

One third of the *most cited* clinical research has replication problems. This means the study cannot be replicated with similar results!! WOW!! I thought this seemed to be a very large number, but it wasn't as large as the vast majority of other, less-cited clinical research. If the study cannot be replicated; what does this say about the study? Yet, we are paying for and taking all of these medications? You have got to be kidding. Where are the regulations they are required to follow before a drug passes FDA approval? Let's dig into this a little further.

Dr. Ioannidis found, despite the fact that 45 of the 49 most cited articles he studied provided methods to verify the effectiveness of their respective claims, 41% of them were shown to be wrong or grossly exaggerated.[21, 22]

Think about what that means. Out of the 49 most cited medical research articles, 45 of them provided the methods to replicate the study. Okay, why didn't all 49 provide the methods, but let that go for a minute. 41% of them could not be replicated!!! You have got to be kidding!! But they got through the FDA? And our physicians are prescribing them?

When I told my wife, Mary, about this, she just shook her head. "Who do they think they are, that they can pawn all of this nonsense onto the MDs and then the MDs pawn it onto us. I thought this was supposed to be hard science, that they actually knew what they were doing or prescribing. Why isn't this stuff all over the evening news and in the newspapers?"

By the way, Mary wrote a book for the Entwined Collection as well: *Arthritis: Manage It or Eliminate It.*

The challenge is, Mary was right. Why isn't it? Would you believe when I went to some of the MDs, they actually accused me of believing in the "Conspiracy Theory" that Conventional Western Medicine was a scam.

I was dumbfounded. Were the MDs really that ignorant of what was going on? Was it all MDs? What about the ones who were not ignorant, what did they do with the information?

Neither Mary or I had the answers to these questions so Mary pushed me to expand my research even further. I went back to my drawing board.

I started to ask whether the physicians understand what is going on, and then asked myself to what degree do the scientists understand what is going on.

Once again, I was disappointed with what I found.

Several studies have revealed that scientists are aware of the misconduct amongst their peers but do not report it!! 40% of surveyed researchers were aware of misconduct and 17% of clinical trial researchers personally knew of fabricated data.[23] Another source claims: "only around 50% of all trials conducted by pharmaceutical companies is actually published and released for review by the scientific community. According to the Wall Street Journal, only 41% of over 600 studies sponsored by the National Institute of Health (NIH) were published within 3 years of completion."[24]

It would appear that not only are scientists aware of the misconduct but the research showing all the negative outcomes is simply not published. They only publish the positive results. This would lead the FDA to approve a drug that shouldn't be approved and lead physicians to prescribe a drug that could be detrimental! Is that why so many drugs end up getting recalled.

Marketing
Marketing is another big issue with medical research. The marketing of a drug doesn't just involve how it is

marketed to physicians, but also how it is marketed to us, the general public.

As far as the general public is concerned, we are exposed to marketing headlines that are very misleading. For instance, "Do Polyphenols Cause Cancer?" When you read the article, they might repeatedly state Polyphenols do not cause cancer. As we all know the headline catches people's attention, the problem is this type of marketing is used both with the general public and the health practitioners.

Unfortunately, Big Pharma carefully constructs the information given to the drug company representatives (which are typically English graduates – not biochemists, researchers or anything to do with medicine or research). This information is carefully designed to encourage the physicians to prescribe their drugs. The same occurs with conferences and other presentations given by physicians, drug company representatives and others to physicians.

I was talking with one physician about a new medication being prescribed for seniors who are constipated. The physician had just come away from a medical conference where the drug was presented as safe and reliable without side effects. Yet, I had already found three sites identifying class action law suits against the drug. The physician had not looked for any indicators against the drug, but rather had simply accepted what Big Pharma had presented.

Unfortunately, this blind acceptance about Big Pharma and what they promote is the general rule of thumb amongst most physicians.

Further, there is a terrific amount of investigation concerning MDs and professors who are paid to provide presentations based on false or inaccurate data. According to the CaliforniaHealthLine.org website, California physicians have received $28.6 million from the major drug companies to market/promote their products over just a few years. According to ProPublica, an independent, non-profit newsroom that produces investigative journalism in the public interest, the amount nationwide is increased to $281.9 million. This does not include drug samples. In addition, physicians are offered opportunities to travel with their families for continuing education, are given gifts of various value as well as discounts and meals brought to the physician's offices.[25] This same article states that 290 physicians have faced disciplinary action or other sanctions in various states.

Remember, Big Pharma want the MDs to prescribe their medications. So, they tell the MDs only what they want the MDs to know.

Dr. Ioannidis' claims:

> He and his team have shown, again and again, and in many different ways, that much of what biomedical researchers conclude in published studies and conclusions that doctors keep in mind

when they prescribe antibiotics or blood-pressure medication, or when they advise us to consume more fiber or less meat, or when they recommend surgery for heart disease or back pain is misleading, exaggerated, and **often flat-out wrong.** He charges as much as 90 percent of the published medical information that doctors rely on is flawed.[26]

Imagine that, 90% of the published medical information physicians rely on is flawed. But it is this very misleading information that guides MDs to prescribe a medication for given symptom!!

How do you feel about that? Does that disturb you as much as it does me?

We, the general public, are paying out billions of dollars annually for drugs based on flawed research? These drugs deplete the body of nutrients and cause cancer and strokes and heart attacks and acidosis and, and, and!!! Absolutely unbelievable! And the physicians just keep pumping out the prescriptions!!

Chapter 4
Relative Risk Versus Absolute Risk

Here we go again. I have never taken a course on research or design, or statistics. But as I said earlier, I am familiar with the line, "Figures don't lie till statisticians start to figure," and now I was getting more and more interested in this stuff.

I had to learn enough that I could explain it to Mary and if I passed the test there, then I was willing to put it in the book. There was much that I didn't understand well enough to explain, so I left it out. In addition, I needed to keep the book short enough as most readers would not want to read the volumes and volumes I could have addressed.

My next step was to make an appointment with Dr. Daniel from the Gibson Clinic. He has a PhD in nutrition and does a lot of actual research with nutrients and body function. I asked him if I could take him out for lunch and pick his brain. Dr. Daniel laughed and agreed. We decided on Friday, it was going to be a slow day as he only had a conference meeting with a couple of international laboratories. It worked great for me; we agreed on a restaurant and a time.

I walked into the restaurant a little early. I wanted to set up my laptop and get prepared before Dr. Daniel came in, but Dr. Daniel was already there and waved me over to the window table he was sitting at.

"Hi there Papa Johnny, I hope you don't mind sitting here. I brought my laptop and have been doing some research while I waited for you. This is a great spot for the Wi-Fi. How are you doing?"

"Here I thought I was going to be early and have time to set up before you got here. Apart from that, I am doing great." I responded.

"No problem. Sit down and get yourself organized while I finish off this paper I'm working on. There is a menu if you want or you can start by ordering yourself a drink."

I sat down and got myself organized. There was plenty of room for both of our laptops and still enough room for our lunch plates when we ordered. We both ordered a tea. I followed Dr Daniel's lead when ordering and had a beautiful baked salmon, rice pilaf and Greek salad. I thought privately that it might be a boring lunch with a Dr of Nutrition, but it turned out to be a beautiful lunch.

"So, you want to know about how MDs are manipulated with statistics," Dr. Daniel led the way into the conversation.

"You got it. I hear the saying, 'Figures don't lie until statisticians start to figure,' but how can you make figures lie?"

"Okay, a more general response is that there are just so many ways, it is unreal. Let's just look at one type of distortion, Relative Risk versus Absolute Risk. This is a big one, and it totally misleads both the MDs and the patients.

Let's look at one example: the claims that blood pressure medications cut the risk of a stroke by about 40%. One would naturally make the assumption the drug prevents strokes in 400 people out 1000 people per year. But that isn't the case at all. The actual data shows about 15 out of a 1000 people, with mild hypertension, will have a stroke over the next 5 years. If we put all 1000 people on the medication, then the number of 15 will drop down to 9, out of a 1000, over a period of 5 years.

A drop from 15 strokes down to 9 strokes is a relative 40% drop that will occur over 5-year duration. This is called a Relative Risk Reduction. But the Actual Risk Reduction is a reduction of one stroke per year out of a 1000. This is a significant difference from the 400 a year that the marketing implies. The Actual Risk is significantly below 1%.

So, with all the people on this unnecessary prescription, we have to ask the question: what are the symptoms that the other 994 people put on the drugs are likely to suffer? Well, those blood pressure medications can actually increase other heart problems and even cause death. They cause a depletion of vital minerals in the body, things like fatigue and dizziness or loss of sexual function, and things like digestive disorders, anxiety and restlessness, anemia, cough, and other issues.

Yet, hypertension can be resolved with diet, hydration and walking, which is not only kinder to the body but also kinder to the pocket book.

Now according to the Cochrane Collaboration, the anti-hypertensive drugs do NOT help those with mild hypertension. AND, the data also shows the majority of those with hypertension that are put on prescription drugs, only have mild hypertension and do not benefit from the medications.[27]

Does that make sense to you?"

I simply nodded my head while I typed my notes.

Dr Daniel carried on, "Let's look at it in a different way, statistics can be misleading. The statistics for statin drugs, that are used for high cholesterol, are also very misleading.

The whole cholesterol issue is a problem in and of itself. Too little cholesterol is far more dangerous than too high cholesterol. Most physicians don't know that there are many types of HDL (claimed to be the good cholesterol) and even more types of LDL. In fact, if HDL 3a is higher than 2b or 2c, you are in deep trouble. I can go on and on about the different types of cholesterol. Never mind why cholesterol is so needed in the body.

Anyways, back to the topic on hand. The claim is the drugs reduce the risk of heart attacks by 33%. Sounds good, doesn't it?

But what are the actual figures? Out of a 100 people, 3 people are likely to have a heart attack. If we put all 100 people on the prescription drug, that number drops to 2. The reduction of 3 heart attacks down to 2 heart attacks is a reduction of 33%. That is the Relative Risk Reduction. The Absolute Risk Reduction is one less person out of a 100! Which is significantly below 1%.

So again, what are the side effects the remaining 99 people might have to deal with? These side effects become the symptoms used to determine the next drug you are going to get prescribed. Statin drugs cause a significant decrease in CoQ10. Statin drugs paralyze the last enzyme required to make cholesterol in the body, thus preventing the body from making cholesterol. Further down the chain, beyond making cholesterol is where the synthesis of CoQ10 takes place. Why is this important? The CoQ10 compound is required in every cell of the body to make fuel. With the loss of CoQ10, anything and everything can go wrong. The primary symptoms people experience are muscle aches and pain and deterioration, immune issues, pancreatic and liver issues which can lead to diabetes and other problems, cognitive and memory issues, as well as sexual dysfunction, cataracts and anemia.

Yet, not only is the whole cholesterol issue totally false, but even if there are cholesterol issues, we can easily solve it with real food and herbs that help the body regulate cholesterol production. These have only positive benefits and no negative side effects. Unfortunately, food and herbs do not support Big Pharma.

Let's stop for a moment while I get more hot water for my tea." Dr. Daniel signalled for the waitress, "Do you want anything else?"

"This is rather funny. I never would have enjoyed this kind of lunch historically. Today, I look forward to eating this kind of healthy meal. But no, I don't need anything else.

I hope you know how much I appreciate all your help with understanding this information. I had no idea physicians were so manipulated. And the bigger problem is, not only do the rest of us not know how manipulated they are, but the physicians don't know either. The whole medical system seems such a racket. I don't know how we allowed it to get so bad. I guess I will find out as I work through this book."

The waitress came and filled up the tea pots and asked if we needed anything else. It didn't take long before Dr. Daniel started again. His passion about this stuff was apparent; he loved talking about it even if it was to someone as ignorant of all this stuff as me. I enjoyed listening to him, if for no other reason, then to listen to his passion that came through loud and clear.

"Let's use another example. The elderly are often put on prescriptions for osteoporosis. Unfortunately, what the drugs do is simply paralyze the osteoclasts. There are two primary types of bone cells, osteoblasts and osteoclasts. The osteoblasts are responsible for maintaining, repairing and remodelling your bones. The osteoclasts are responsible for eliminating the by-products created through this process.

With the osteoclasts paralyzed, they cannot eliminate the by-products. So, any increased density is simply made up of garbage by-products, not strong healthy bones. If the osteoclasts cannot do their job, the bones become even more brittle and susceptible to breaking even though they are considered 'denser'.

The Relative Risk Reduction tells us the risk of fracture drops by 50% when people take the prescription. The number of fractures dropped from 2.2% to 1.1% of the whole population. Definitely this looks like a 50% drop.

The Actual Risk Reduction is 22 people out of a 1000, versus 11 people of a 1000. Only 22 people out of a

1000 would experience a problem and that number drops to 11 out of a 1000 if all 1000 people take the drug. Again, the Actual Risk Reduction is less than 1%.

So once again, what are the risks of taking the drug? The osteoclasts cannot function, the bones fill up with garbage, and people are actually more susceptible to bone fractures. But they did help support Big Pharma's bottom line." Dr. Daniel provided me with a number of websites explaining this nicely and easily, so I would have a backup for the book. I am glad he did.[28, 29, 30]

"Now, what can we do if we help the same people with REAL Medicine? First of all, we **won't** put them on calcium supplements. Most people do not need calcium supplements. In fact, too much calcium in the blood can also cause more problems with abnormal heart rhythms, calcifications, and injuries in the esophagus and stomach.

In the bones, calcium is a competitor and prevents the bones from absorbing the minerals the bones actually need. And of course, more and more research is coming out with how detrimental the synthetic supplements Big Pharma provides are.

However, we also have to be careful here, because there are a lot of synthetics in the nutraceuticals as well. So, we identify what the body needs or has too much of, in terms of minerals like boron, copper, magnesium, manganese, potassium, selenium, silicon, sodium, strontium, vanadium, zinc and vitamins like D3 & K2.

When we make sure the proper ratios of the different minerals and vitamins and other nutrients are in the body, there is only positive side-effects and no negative ones.

Once again, REAL medicine eliminates the underlying issues whereas synthetic medicine contributes to and even exacerbates the problem."

"Wow, that is a lot of information." My fingers were typing as fast I could. I was sure glad I had been taking notes. Once I caught up, I took a sip of tea and asked the question that had been dying to ask, "do the MDs really *not* know this stuff?"

Dr Daniel carried on. "You are right Papa Johnny. Most MDs have no idea of the difference between Absolute Risk and Relative Risk. There are a few studies that have revealed that when physicians are taught the difference between relative and absolute risk, with regard to a given prescription, their prescription rates drop dramatically. So of course, Big Pharma doesn't tell them.

I would suggest that, in general, MDs don't knowingly mislead their patients. I would like to believe that most physicians went into medicine to help people. The problem is, they are being mislead too."

"Are there other kinds of issues distorting data results that I should be looking into?" I pushed for more information.

"Of course, there are all kinds of issues. Not only are the medical sciences full of fraud, but there are a variety of other problems. For instance, studies that were signed off yet never even done, negative results getting filed away and only positive results being published or reported to the FDA, and the problems go on and on. More and more of these kinds of thing are getting reported and some of it actually gets to the internet, which is a good thing.

But other kinds of issues arising are with the analysis itself. Most of medical research uses simple correlational analysis or multivariate analysis (MANOVA analysis) when they should be using complex Canonical analysis. Unfortunately, those kinds of analysis are even more expensive and time consuming and of course, finances are always an issue."

"I have only just started learning about the different types of statistical analysis. The ones I have written about so far include correlational, MANOVAs and Canonicals. Can you give me the 'Definition for Dummies' version?"

"I am impressed. You have been doing your research. Ok, let's give it a try. A Correlational Analysis simply determines if two variables occur together. As one increases the other either decreases, doesn't change, or increases as well. They may have no causal relationship whatsoever. But they do have a strong positive correlation. A good example of an inappropriate correlational process being incorrectly identified as a causal relationship is: suggesting that the sun coming up causes people to wake up. When in fact, while there there is a good correlational relationship, the cause for getting up could be: the alarm going off, children waking up, needing to go the bathroom, etc. These things tend to happen in the morning but neither one causes the other to happen.

This is a big problem with a lot of medical research. For instance, some cholesterol counts increase with age which usually has nothing to do with your diet, but rather, the body is using cholesterol to patch up bleeds in the arteries and veins. This type of healing occurs daily in all of us, but takes longer to complete as we get older. Consequently, the liver, provides more LDL cholesterol to patch up the bleeds. The cholesterol is not the problem, the bleed is."

"So, like you guys keep saying, cholesterol is like the fireman at the fire, it is not causing the fire. So, while they both tend to happen together, firemen go to fires, the firemen are not causing the fire."

"There you got it," Dr. Daniel smiled at my response. "Now when we are talking about a MANOVA analysis, we are analyzing two or more dependent variables with an independent variable. How does change in one variable affect the other variable(s) when a third variable remains constant?

The difference between a MANOVA and a Canonical Analysis is Canonical Analysis looks at the relationships between several factors, each of which has several variables. Canonicals also work with predictor variables and criterion variables. Again, this is a more costly analysis – so they don't like doing them.

But let's give you a simple example. Factor 1 could be called "exercise" and the variables could be: the levels of exercise, types of exercise, duration of exercise, intensity of exercise. Factor 2 could be called "diet", and the variables might include: vegetarian, paleo, Mediterranean. Then we would combine the different variables both within and between the factors and look at what effect they had on the resulting pulse rate.

When we are dealing with the body and all of the biochemical interactions, we need to use this kind of analysis. Why? Because everything is so interactive with everything else. But, once again, most medical research does not do this kind of analysis.

Let's try to summarize all of this for you. There are five components of a study that are hugely important.

Is the hypothesis made on grounded evidence or is the hypothesis faulty to begin with? This is becoming more and more of an issue with the Western Conventional medical sciences.

The design of a study whether it is a double blind, cross over, cross over double blind, randomized controlled trials, etc.

The number of subjects involved, how they are recruited, who stays in, who leaves, and why they leave.

The type of analysis used. Simply put, whether it is a correlational, manova or canonical, although there are other types of analysis.

How the results are marketed. The one issue we looked at was the relative risk versus the actual risk, but there are all kinds of other issues here too, including whether or not the negative results are even reported.

Issues can and do occur at every step of the process."

"I am not sure what to say at this point, Dr. Daniel. My belly may be full, but my head is definitely overwhelmed. The fact that way too many physicians don't even know this stuff is beyond scary. How do any of us know who to believe and who not to believe? I used to think physicians simply didn't know about what nutrients the body required and I thought that was huge. But apparently, they don't even know what is behind the stuff they are taught! Why is it you guys know all this stuff, when they don't?"

"Good question Papa Johnny. The simple answer is they are governed by Big Pharma. Big Pharma determines most of the criterion for med schools, determines the protocol and procedures the MDs have to follow, and control the continuing education the MDs get.

On the other hand, practitioners in all the different REAL medicine modalities are not controlled by Big Pharma.

It is unfortunate, that in some are areas, the naturopaths have fought for and received licence to prescribe some drug. This is contradictory considering that naturopaths claim prescription drugs are toxic. But in addition, it has also left them open to Big Pharma control.

Having said that, just because they operate in different healing modalities doesn't mean they keep up to date on all of the recent research. Nor does it mean they really understand research, design and analysis either.

Where they do benefit, is they have to take course work in Western medicine. Many of the programs require the students take at least 2,000 hours of Western medicine theory in the first two years, which is exactly what the med school students have to take. The difference is the REAL Medicine programs also teach nutrition, herbal medicine, acupuncture, homeopathy, etc. depending on what they are focused on. They, in effect, get a lot more training than the MDs do."

"So, the short and the long of it is Big Pharma rules and MDs are legalized drug pushers for the Big Guys?"

Dr Daniel just smiled.

I was more determined than ever to get the message out there. I couldn't wait to get home and start putting my book together. I wanted everyone, including the MDs to know what they were up against.

Chapter 5
Cardiology

The two major causes of death are heart and cancer issues. So, I thought I would look at those two fields of medicine in more depth. I found that these were also the most commonly discussed issues on the internet.

I decided to start researching issues regarding the heart. The two most interesting and commonly discussed cardio issues were cholesterol and blood pressure.

I thought I should start my research by interviewing a few cardiologists and, of course, the practitioners at the Gibson Clinic, to give me their ideas about the two topics. I made an appointment with the family physician to get a referral to a cardiologist, but I had to wait for a month.

In the meantime, I went to the Gibson Clinic; they were trained in both Conventional Medicine and REAL Medicine, whereas the cardiologists are only trained in Conventional Medicine. I made an appointment with the Gibson Clinic and explained to the receptionist it would be helpful to have a conference with all the practitioners as I was doing a research project on cholesterol and blood pressure. Dr. Jane phoned me back and suggested we book time on a Friday evening. They didn't normally book clients at that time and everyone could be present. I was really appreciative of them taking the time and asked if it would be okay if my wife Mary, daughter Maria and her husband Duncan all came along. The Clinic knew my family.

Although it was my book and research, I knew they would all be very interested in listening to the discussion. Dr. Jane laughed and said of course. As part of the 'Entwined Book Club', she knew what we were all up to and suggested we turn it into a potluck dinner and have some fun with it. We confirmed the date and time and hung up.

When I got off the phone, I turned to my wife and with a broad smile on my face and confirmed, "That Dr. Jane is one incredible person. Do you know she organized it, so we can all go over for a potluck dinner and everyone can take part in my interview? This is great because you guys can all help me come up with questions I need to explore."

Mary smiled, "I think she also has a soft spot for you. How many physicians would take the time to provide you with that kind of information?" I went back to the drawing board and organized a list of questions I wanted to ask. I wanted to come across as a professional and knew I had some homework to do.

Maria and Duncan readily agreed to the potluck. As usual, they wanted to learn as much as they could. Duncan drove the four of us over to the Clinic on Friday night and the receptionist guided us into the board room. Dr. Jane, or someone, had already put out plates and cutlery. We put our dinner contributions on the table, seated ourselves and waited for the Gibsons to come in. Pappy came in first.

"Hello everyone. How is everyone tonight?" he asked as he put a casserole on the table. Before anyone had a chance to speak Dr. Daniel and Dr. Jane appeared, and everyone was hugging everyone.

Dr. Jim wondered in, "Hi everyone. This is going to be an interesting dinner. Julie can't make it till late. She is on a long-distance call with a practitioner in Germany. But we should all get started."

As plates were handed out and dishes passed around, Pappy started the discussion. "Well this should be fun. So, Papa Johnny is writing a political book. You are going to call it the "*Politics of Medicine*, correct? And from what I understand you want to get everyone's opinion on the Cholesterol Myth tonight?"

"Yes, you hit it right on. Although already I changed the name of the book to: *A Politics of Western Medicine*. I thought that might be more accurate.

I thought I would start with the more specialized investigations dealing with blood pressure and cholesterol. And, as usual, I thought I would listen to your perspective first as all of you have training in both Conventional Western medicine and in your individualized special fields of REAL medicine.

I want to thank you for such a great idea, this potluck dinner with all the practitioners and with Mary, Maria and Duncan. They say two heads are better than one, so this must be a great group.

Do you mind if we start by defining what exactly cholesterol does in the body? What makes it so bad?"

The Gibsons all started to smile.

"Well, first off Papa Johnny, cholesterol is NOT bad. In fact, the body could not function without cholesterol. Cholesterol is essential to life." Dr. Jim started and nodded to Dr. Jane to continue.

"Your body needs cholesterol in the membrane of every one of your millions of cells. The cholesterol in the cellular membranes helps regulate the membrane fluidity so only the appropriate compounds can be transported in and out of the cell. Otherwise toxins may be transported into the cell or conversely toxins may not get excreted from the cell.

Your millions of neurons also need cholesterol to make up the myelin material that insulates them. It is required for normal synapse and dendrite (receptor) formation which allows messages to move throughout the brain and the nervous system. In fact, the brain uses about 20% of the body's cholesterol.

Your body uses cholesterol for other things as well. For instance, cholesterol is used to make all the steroid hormones, the sex hormones, adrenal hormones, the corticosteroids, to help make Vitamin D, and of course, it is used to make all the different HDLs and LDLs and VLDLs, etc.

One important cholesterol function, especially as the body gets older, is to patch up arterial bleeds. If the body cannot patch a bleed fast enough, the liver sends out extra cholesterol to patch up the bleed, so we don't bleed to death. Western medical research operates on the hypothesis that cholesterol plaque causes heart disease, when in fact, the cholesterol is like the fireman at the fire. The cholesterol is solving the problem not causing it; a huge difference."

Dr Daniel winked at me as we had already discussed this. I nodded but wanted the others to hear what I had already been told.

Dr Jane continued, "Your liver also turns cholesterol into the bile that goes through your gallbladder and into your small intestine to help break down the fats from your meal, so the enzymes can work with them to metabolize and absorb them. The bile is also required to absorb Vitamins like A, D, E, & K." Dr. Jane nodded to Dr. Daniel to continue.

"The whole issue about getting too much cholesterol in your diet is pretty much a falsehood. Because cholesterol is so important to the body, the liver makes 75-80% of your cholesterol and regulates how much needs to be made in response to how much is in your diet. Even if you get none in your diet, your liver will make it. If you get too much in your diet, the body can down regulate it in one of three ways. One, the liver can simply make less of it. Two, the liver can convert more of it into bile and eliminate it with the stools. Three, the colon will absorb less of it. So, with a proper healthy diet, there is no need to be concerned about too much cholesterol.

In fact, in 2010, the guidelines put before the FDA recommended taking cholesterol foods off the "no-no list"!! Diet cholesterol is no longer a villain!! Although, unfortunately, saturated fats are still on the list. Oh well, one slow step at a time for the MDs."

"Well then, why do we hear all this stuff about too much LDL and needing to take statin drugs?" I asked.

"Good question, Papa Johnny," Pappy responded, "First of all, all cholesterol is just cholesterol. When they categorize cholesterol like that, it is in reference to what it is attached to. Cholesterol gets attached to other fats and to proteins. There are actually many different types of HDL and LDL. MDs only know about the major categories, the raw numbers or the ratios, which at worst tell us nothing, and at best, are very misleading."[31]

"You see, there are some types of HDL that are harmful. Now I already talked with Papa Johnny about this, so let's see what he remembers." Dr. Daniel directed and nodded at me.

I took a deep breath and gave my best: "If HDL 3 is higher than HDL 2a or 2b, we are in trouble. On the other hand, if we don't get enough of some of the LDLs, we are in trouble. In fact, some of the current research is showing that some of the LDLs are even more important than the HDLs."

"Way to go Papa Johnny. I am impressed. You really were listening." Dr Daniel acknowledged.

I smugly looked at my wife and daughter and Duncan. They were all laughing and very impressed.

Dr. Daniel continued on, "MDs are also concerned about the TGs or the triglycerides. They are linked to both heart disease and diabetes. TGs increase in response to high levels of grains and sugars, lack of exercise, smoking and drinking and yes, they are a concern. Actually, LDLs can be a concern as well, especially when they get oxidized, which is a good reason to make sure you get your anti-oxidants.

The problem, or one of the many problems is, it takes years and years for this basic research to get to the MDs and into the hospitals. Big Pharma, of course, is basically in charge of most of the curriculums, the protocol and the procedures for MDs, plus they are making big money on the statins. Lipitor itself is claimed to make over a billion dollars a day!! So why would they teach anything differently?"

Dr. Jim jumped in, "What about that research you were working on with regard to what the MDs are now saying, Jane?"

"Yes, it is really sad. Historically, or at least since the 50's, LDLs were identified as the bad guys and it was claimed that it builds up in arteries and creates plaque. Dr. William Casteilli was the former director of the Framingham Heart Study. He said in Framingham, Mass., 'the more saturated fat one ate, the more cholesterol one ate, the more calories one ate, the lower the person's serum cholesterol. The opposite of what…Keys et al (the original cholesterol researchers) would predict…We found that people who ate the most cholesterol, ate the most saturated fat, ate the most calories, weighed the least and were the most physically active.'"[32]

"Wow. That goes against everything we ever hear from our MDs and the general media," Maria looked astonished.

"There is a cardiologist who admits he has 25 years of experience and has performed over 5,000 open heart surgeries," Dr. Daniel elaborated, "and now claims that 'The discovery a few years ago that inflammation in the artery wall is the real cause of heart disease is slowly leading to a paradigm shift in how heart disease and other chronic ailments will be treated.'"[33]

Duncan looked really upset, "You mean to tell me it took him 25 years and 5,000 open heart surgeries to figure it out, and he even admits it?"

"Yeah, you're right," Dr. Jane continued, "in the same article he is quoted as saying, 'I saw it in over 5,000 surgical patients spanning 25 years who all shared one common denominator -- inflammation in their arteries.'[34]

I can tell by the looks on your faces that you might be thinking why on earth didn't he say something or do something different before now? Some might want to defend him and say, 'well it got to the point where he had to do open heart surgery.' A good argument if you lack other important information. However, the cardiologist goes on to say, 'By eliminating inflammatory foods and adding essential nutrients from fresh unprocessed food, you will reverse years of damage in your arteries and throughout your body from consuming the typical American diet."[35]

My jaw dropped open and Maria questioned: "He knew it wasn't a matter of cholesterol AND he knew you can reverse it with diet AND he kept on doing open heart surgeries??"

The room fell quiet for a moment as we digested this. After a few minutes I asked: "Jane, from what you implied, it sounds like he is close to retiring?"

Dr. Jane nodded. "I find it interesting that he is coming out and acknowledging this after. he has already made his millions at a great physical and financial cost to his patients. Is there an ethical concern here?"

"It gets worse," Dr. Jane continued, "he also acknowledged 'The injury and inflammation in our blood vessels is caused by the low-fat diet recommended for years by mainstream medicine.'"[36]

"In summary," Grandma Mary had been silent up to now just soaking in all the information, "he not only knew what the MDs, and in particular the cardiologists, were recommending was wrong, but he knew the right recommendation would actually reverse the problem, yet he still chose to do the surgeries?"

I was busy taking notes rather than eating. But I paused and looked up. "There are a number of things I need to figure out. I need to figure out why MDs are told falsehoods about cholesterol. Why is it so misunderstood? Why are MDs told to measure cholesterol and prescribe drugs? How are they compensated for prescribing the drugs?

I know that the anti-cholesterol drugs, or statins, cause all kinds of problems; they block the body's ability to make the much-required cholesterol and, in the process of doing so, block the body's capacity to make the CoQ10 that every cell requires in order to make the fundamental fuel for every cell. Thus, the side effects can be almost anything and everything, as nothing can happen without the fuel."

"I see that you are busy writing down lots of notes Papa Johnny, but there is another huge component you need to understand. Jane, would you please explain to this group the massive number of negative side effects of statin drugs?" Dr. Jim directed.

"This is really important. Every cell of the body requires fuel to function. Hundreds, if not thousands, of functions in occur in every cell, depending on the complexity of the cell. The part of the cell creating the fuel is the mitochondria. The number of mitochondria in a given cell is directly related to the cell's requirement for fuel. Consequently, heart and brain cells have upwards of 2500 mitochondria, all producing fuel for the cells.

How does this relate to the statin drugs? Well statin drugs prevent the body from making an important compound necessary for the mitochondria to make that fuel, CoQ10. Without CoQ10, the cells cannot make fuel and subsequently, everything starts to go sideways into dysfunction, cancer or cellular death.

Consequently, statin drugs can cause everything from muscle aches, pain and atrophy to general fatigue to loss of cognitive function. Basically, anything and everything can go wrong." Dr Jane paused and looked around the group to make sure everyone was following her explanation.

"So, if this is all true, then why are MDs required to prescribe statin drugs?" Maria thought she knew the answer but needed to ask anyway.

"Well as we all know, money is the driver of Big Pharma. They have no moral or ethical responsibility to our health, but they do have a legal obligation to make money for their shareholders. That is why, when we are looking at the research, we always start by looking at who is funding the study," Dr. Daniel explained.

"Well, don't the MDs and cardiologists do that?" Grandma Mary wanted to know.

"Well, no, not necessarily. For starters, most physicians are not trained in research, design and analysis. Even when they look at studies, it is usually just at the Abstract and/or the Conclusion or Summary. Even if they do understand the different types of research design and analysis, they are probably not going to take the time to read the research and if they actually go that far, they are pretty unlikely to look at who funded the study," Dr. Jane said with a grimace.

"We can go further than that. Even if they actually took the time to do all the reading and they understand research dilemmas and issue, never mind who funded the study and how it might have been biased, there are very few who are willing to stand up and question the accepted dogma." Dr. Jim said with a sigh, "Unfortunately, that doesn't just apply to medicine, but rather it applies to all the sciences from psychology to physics.

Students are taught what the system wants them to know. There are few professions where students are actually pushed, encouraged and taught to go outside the given boundaries and accepted dogmas. Students are not encouraged to challenge the "Old Men's Club". MDs are taught how to manage symptoms, not eliminate the underlying issues. As a consequence, unless a practitioner is truly interested in his clients and wants to eliminate the underlying issues, follows through with their progress, has the intelligence to question the status quo and has the confidence to stand up to the system, he/she will simply follow along with the status quo."

"So, do you try to lower cholesterol?" I asked.

"We take the approach the body is wiser than we are. So, what we do is determine if the body needs help to regulate the cholesterol. We will use diet and herbs that help the body to establish the regulation it needs. We also look at whether the mitochondria are working properly, whether the body has enough CoQ10, and are the cellular methylation cycles working? There are a number of issues that need to be determined before any action is taken.

In fact, the way we look at it is, low cholesterol is actually more of a problem than high cholesterol. In addition, the research is quite clear: a hard, tart apple a day and walking a mile a day actually does more good for the body than the statin drugs," Dr. Jane responded.[37]

"So how does cholesterol connect with high blood pressure?" Papa Johnny pushed.

Dr. Jim started passing the dinner offerings around the table again as he answered, "Cholesterol is connected with high blood pressure in a couple of ways. If there is plaque, inflammation or anything else that narrows the arteries and/or veins, it is going to put pressure on the heart to pump harder to get that blood around the body. That is part of the problem.

The old hypothesis is *all* narrowing of the arteries is caused from cholesterol plaque. Current research actually shows that there are all kinds of issues that can cause inflammation which can cause high blood pressure. A variety of different types of toxins can cause inflammation, oxidized cholesterol can cause inflammation, calcification can cause both inflammation and hardening of the arteries which is hard on the heart.

Then there are issues like improper insulin and leptin signaling that can cause arterial inflammation. Additional huge issues revolve around sugars and

AGEs (Advanced Glycation Endproducts) which can cause damage to the arteries."

"What are AGEs?" Grandma Mary wanted to know.

"When there are excess sugars, the body will link sugar with either fats or proteins causing AGEs without the direction of enzymes. There are many important sugar compounds called glycoproteins (sugar linked with protein) and glycolipids (sugar linked with fat). The difference between the AGEs and these important glycoproteins and glycolipids are the latter are designed by enzymes. The AGEs made in the body without the direction of enzymes are dangerous. They attach to the sides of arteries, or any other cellular structures in the body, and cause a variety of different types of damage." Dr. Daniel explained, "When the cellular structure of arteries, or veins, is damaged, inflammation occurs. Inflammation blocks the flow of blood. Pressure is put on the heart. Blood pressure increases."

"Other issues can also cause high blood pressure. If we don't make enough nitric oxide, it is difficult for the arteries to expand and contract which puts more pressure on the heart and increases blood pressure. If the kidneys are not working effectively, the kidneys can't extract extra fluids and substances from the blood which makes the blood thick and heavy to push, which puts more pressure on the heart. The kidneys may not be working effectively for a number of reasons.

The problem is all the different types of blood pressure medications deplete the body of nutrients like magnesium and potassium. In fact, most drugs, whether they are over the counter drugs or prescription drugs, deplete the body of nutrients. Unfortunately, when physicians are aware of this, they prescribe synthetic nutrients to help replenish the body. Unfortunately, this makes matters even worse because, as we have said, the synthetic nutrients are more of a detriment than a benefit to the body," Dr. Jane elaborated.

At that point Julie walked in. "Hi Hon, how did the phone call go?" Dr. Jim asked his wife.

"Helping out an MD in Germany. He worked on my time schedule because I was helping him. I think we got it all figured out. How is everything going here? Are you getting the information you are looking for Papa Johnny?"

"Well, I think the information I am getting is creating more questions than answers. I can't believe Western medicine is so screwed up."

"It is, and it is too bad. So many MDs went to med school believing they were going to be able to help people and they have no idea how much harm they are causing. So many are taught to believe in western pharmaceuticals, they assume anything that goes against Big Pharma is simply part of the "Conspiracy Theory".

What can you do? Despite the challenges, we see our responsibility is in helping in our clients learn, we provide programs on the internet, radio and in the community, and we write books and articles.

When it comes to the physicians, we attempt to guide them to the ton of research right there in front of their noses. If they remain blinded by what Big Pharma taught them in med school and continues to push down their throats with the drug reps and the 'Continuing Education' programs they put on, then we have to take a deep breath and let it be. The rewarding component is that more and more MDs are waking up to the fact that Western Medicine is not the be all and end all it is claimed to be.

But where were you in the conversation before I walked in?" Julie sat down and started to dish herself a plate of food.

"Well overall this meeting was about cholesterol and blood pressure. Ultimately, Papa Johnny wanted to get a good base of understanding of cholesterol and blood pressure. And then I suppose you want to find some good places to start doing your research?" Dr. Jim questioned me.

"Yes, that would be great. Where should I go from here?" I really wanted to know where I needed to go next.

"Well some of the places you can start with are, PubMed and PLoS. Personally, I prefer PLoS which stands for the People's Library of Sciences. As you start doing your research you will come across names like: Dr. Lipman, Dr. Rosedale, Dr. Stephen Sinatra, and Dr. Chris Kresser. You may want to research the Cochrane Collaboration, an independent global network of researchers, professionals, etc. interested in health. People see them as the critical gatekeepers of medical research, so to speak. They are supposed to set the standard for the evaluation of healthcare interventions. On the other hand, Dr. Bero found "only 46 out of 151 Cochrane drug treatment reviews analyzed reported information on the funding sources of their included studies, and just one-fifth of the reviews provided the funding sources for all their studies. Further, only about 1 in 10 reviews provided information on whether study authors had financial ties to, or were employed by, the pharmaceutical industry."[38]

It doesn't matter where you go, there are huge problems in the system. Historically, you may want to look up Dr. Ancel Keys research and see how flawed it was.

When you look at actual research, always make sure you know who is providing the funding for the study. Always make sure you also use words like conflict, controversies, theories, hypothesis, review, lawsuits, for a start. That way you will get opposing thoughts."

"Well I sure appreciate all the information you have given me. It provokes more questions than it answers, but I guess that's a good thing. I feel overwhelmed, but at the same time, I am feeling a burning desire to get some answers. Thank you so much for all the information that you have provided me."

I put my hands together at my chest in the East Indian fashion. I knew Dr. Jane did this to show recognition and appreciation and I really wanted her and the others to know how much I appreciated them.

They continued to talk while they finished off the food. The discussion was fun and animated, ranging well beyond the scope of cholesterol and high blood pressure. But I was itching to go home and get back to my computer. I had so many more questions I wanted to research now and more direction to start exploring my next topic, cancer.

Chapter 6
Cancer

"In poring over medical journals, he was struck by how many findings of all types were refuted by later findings. Of course, medical-science 'never minds' are hardly secret. And they sometimes make headlines, as when in recent years large studies or growing consensuses of researchers concluded that mammograms, colonoscopies, and PSA tests are far less useful cancer detection tools than we had been told..."[39]

Okay, I learned you don't have to go far to find the FDA gave tests cancer screening tests like the mammograms and PSAs (prostate specific antigen) a "D" rating. Was this 'fail' rating based on new research? No, the decision to change the rating was based on research they have had for eons. Again, I wasn't impressed.

Dr. Mercola wrote about a Boston University cancer scientist, Sheng Wang, who fabricated his findings. Unfortunately, other important studies based their work on those fabricated findings. Now, 10 years of work have gone down the drain.[40] In addition, in reference to cancer research, Dr. Mercola states, "Much of the support comes from flawed and biased 'research' studies that support the use of expensive drugs as detailed in the featured articles."[41]

Although Sheng Wang was required to retract his papers, the fabricated data is likely to live on. In 2001, 22 papers required retraction; in 2006, 139 papers were retracted; in 2011, 339 papers were retracted. I thought Maybe going to the medical journals isn't the wisest move? But I kept going with my research.

There are conflicting claims as to whether Linus Pauling stated the following: "Everyone should know that most cancer research is largely a fraud, and the major cancer research organizations are derelict in their duties to the people who support them."[42]

It's a powerful quote, but I had got into the habit of questioning the quotes and data and references I found on the internet. Although the quote has been referenced over 500 times, the website Paulingblog.com questioned its validity. They claim Linus Pauling did question the Mayo Clinic research and biased data but provided a different quote, "The Mayo article is misleading and dishonest. It might be described as fraudulent. It was purported to be a repetition of Dr. Cameron's study, but it was greatly different, in a way that the Mayo clinic investigators succeeded in hiding from the readers of their paper."[43]

On the other hand, Dr. John Bailer, who apparently was part of the National Cancer Institute staff for 20 years, publicly stated:

> My overall assessment is that the national cancer program must be judged a qualified failure. Our whole cancer research in the past 20 years has been a total failure...When government officials point to survival figures and say they are winning the war against cancer, they are using those survival rates improperly.[44]

Further down the above referenced article is even more disturbing information.

> In fact, some analysts consider that the cancer industry is sustained by a policy of deliberately facing in the wrong direction...concluded that these institutions had become self-perpetuating organisations whose survival depended on the state of no cure. *(They wrote)* a solution to cancer would mean the termination of research programs, the obsolescence of skills, the end of drams of personal glory, triumph over cancer would dry up contributions of self-perpetuating charities and cut off funding from Congress, it would mortally threaten the present clinical establishments by rendering obsolete the expensive surgical, radiological and chemotherapeutic treatments in which so much money, training and equipment is invested. Such fear, however unconscious, may

result in resistance and hostility to alternative approaches in proportion as they are therapeutically promising.[45]

I couldn't believe what I was reading. I read it a few times to make sure I had it right. Basically, it is saying that the cancer industry (Big Pharma, researchers, and oncologists) doesn't want to cure cancer. The cancer industry makes a huge profit and supports a ton of jobs through research and treatment, never mind the support Big Pharma provides to universities for research.

Holy crap! It also suggests that they know various alternative treatments can reverse cancer. In fact, even MDs who have identified simple, effective treatments have been repressed. Unfortunately, many physicians are not aware of this. Hmm. Big Pharma obviously has a lot of control.

I looked in the journal, *Nature*, and found:

> In 2011, several new cancer drugs were approved, built on robust preclinical data. However, the inability of industry and clinical trials to validate results from the majority of publications on potential therapeutic targets suggests a general, systemic problem... we found widespread recognition of this issue...The lack of rigour that currently exists around generation and analysis of preclinical data is reminiscent of the situation in clinical research about 50 years ago.[46]

If there is "widespread recognition of this issue", why isn't something being done?

Secondly, 50 years ago?!?

They knew this stuff that long ago? Oh sh*t.

They are saying that the research on chemotherapy cannot be replicated. Yet, people go through hell on these drugs. There is a huge physical and emotional toll on the body and mind. In addition, many people, especially those without extended benefits or healthcare, go into bankruptcy due to the cost of these drugs.

Why on earth are these drugs being prescribed? Are we all nuts? This system is crazy.

Another issue I found involved cancer research being done on animals. "A large portion of money donated to cancer research by the public is spent on animal research which has, since its inception, been widely condemned as a waste of time and resources."[47]

Wait just a second. Animal research is a waste of time? Why? Animal don't have the same enzyme processes that we do and don't respond in a similar fashion. Just like using horse urine for estrogen that females cannot absorb or using rodents for birth control research when rodents don't have a menstrual cycle.

I don't really like the idea of experimenting on animals but I was under the impression that they were saving lives. So instead, they are still tormenting animals, making them sick. This is cruelty to animals, inhumane and a waste of time and research funds. Why are they still doing it?

I have not been impressed with the fraud, misrepresentation and manipulation of statistics that had discovered, but now they are tormenting animals for no reason. I was starting to really dislike researchers.

I was getting fed up with what I was finding out, so I started to look at the claims about success. It wasn't much better, "…historically, our ability to translate cancer research to clinical success has been remarkably low[1] sadly, clinical trials in oncology have the highest failure rate compared with other therapeutic areas."[48]

The flip side of the coin was even more powerful. I read in the International Agency for Research in Cancer, "80-90% of human cancer is determined environmentally and thus theoretically avoidable".[49] Again, while the quote is often referenced, it is dated back to the 1988.[50] So I kept looking for some more up-to-date information.

The media claimed overall death rates were on the decrease yet, cancer is on the increase with 20,000 people dying of cancer daily. According to the cancer.org website, there will be over 1.6 million new cancer cases diagnosed in 2015 with about 590,000 deaths. Again, the 'war on cancer' has failed miserably.

Okay, at this point I was getting really aggravated. I made an appointment with my family physician to talk about the information I had collected, but he wasn't willing to discuss it at all. He simply evaded my questions with, "that's not my speciality." I asked for an appointment with an oncologist. He wouldn't make the referral because I didn't have cancer.

I was back to the drawing board. Rather than looking at how cancer was not working, I started looking at the finances behind chemotherapy and research. To 'follow the money' as they say. It was apparent Conventional Western medicine cancer treatments only consist of surgery, chemotherapy and radiation. I also found Western medicine costs the typical cancer patient $50,000. An article as of February 2019 stated:

> A new study from academic researchers found that 66.5 percent of all bankruptcies were tied to medical issues —either because of high costs for care or time out of work.[51]

Also, three of the top 50 charities in the US are cancer charities. Some of their employees have salaries over $1 million per year. This is just wrong.

If we look at the finances for Big Pharma, we find quotes like, "…five pharmaceutical companies made a profit margin of 20% or more: Pfizer, Hoffmann-La Roche, AbbVie, GlaxoSmithKline (GSK) and Eli Lilly."[52]

Further research identified that:

> According to these data, the average cost of developing a cancer drug is about $720 million. The average annual revenue is about $2.7 billion. Within just one year, the annual revenue of the top five drugs on this list – which treat lymphoma, prostate, leukemia, and colorectal cancers – covers the total costs of research and development.[53]

Not only is research getting cheaper and cheaper but the cost to the patient is getting bigger and bigger, which leads to bigger wallets for Big Pharma.

I kept exploring. The internet reveals a ton of information.

I found this an interesting quote, "…100 leading oncologists from around the world wrote an open letter in the journal, *Blood*, calling for a reduction in the price of cancer drugs."[54]

I was impressed with the 100 oncologists, but 'p*ss*d off' at the rest when I found out oncologists can make upwards of 80% of their income from the chemotherapy alone! In addition, Big Pharma, in essence, pays out a commission to the physicians with each chemotherapy prescription. This is different from all other prescriptions, wherein the physician has to meet a quota of prescriptions to get the payout.

Professor Paul Workman, the Chief Executive of the Institute for Cancer Research comments on the financial aspect of chemotherapy research, claiming Big Pharma are only interested in those drugs that turn a profit, which of course simply reinforces what we already know. Big Pharma is in *business* to make a *profit*. Any business should be able to turn a profit; we certainly don't have a problem with that, but NOT at the cost of people's health, never mind their financial stability. Workman claims "theoretical scientists have identified 500 cancer related proteins which could be attacked by drugs, but only 5 per cent of these treatments have so far been developed."[55]

"Okay, so we get it. It is all about business and profit. Big Pharma doesn't really care about our health and well-being." I said out loud and Mary caught me.

"Who doesn't care this time?" she asked with interest.

Frustrated with my research, I was happy to talk with Mary. "This time I'm referring to everyone involved in the cancer industry. They know the premises the research is based on are outdated but continue to work with the same hypotheses."

"Come on Johnny, I am sure they are not all bad. They probably went into medicine and research because they wanted to help people. I guess MDs help people directly and researchers either enjoy research or want to help people indirectly. Even if they went into medicine because of family pressure or for some warped sense that it somehow gave them a sense of value, it doesn't make them bad. There are those who get caught up in the process of things. They 'sell their soul' to the company like many lawyers are perceived to do. But just like lawyers, I am sure there are many who have a passion for what they do and have a basic desire to help people. So, don't write them all off. You know as well as I do there are good ones and bad ones in every profession or trade and most are somewhere in between."

Mary was right. I needed to start looking at this whole thing from a different perspective. Maybe if I started to look at things from the other side of the coin. Was there anything REAL medicine could offer?

My first attempts took me to an interesting documentary film called *Cancer: The Forbidden Cures*, albeit it was a little older. The film promotes older known cures like Essiac tea and the Gerson Therapy.

With further research, I found that there are all kinds of REAL medicine treatments for cancer. A tremendous amount of research focused on herbs like turmeric and other plant compounds like beta glycans, curcumoids, betalaines, liminoids, and polyphenols have also been found to reverse cancer.[56] There was all this research identifying numerous treatments that actually helped people and, apparently did a much better job than Western Conventional Medicine.[57, 58]

At this point, I thought I should go and talk with the Gibson Clinic again. Dr. Jane did the most research and worked with the most treatment protocols for cancer. She is a wealth of information. She claims there are several ways to deal with cancer that don't involve harming the body with chemotherapy. Their success rates are significantly better than Conventional medicine. Dr. Jane says that one of her professors claims a 90%+ rate of success across all cancers. WOW!! How come this isn't well known?

I was really looking forward to digging into this favourite topic of Dr Jane's. When Dr. Jane gets started on one of her passion topics, she was simply a pleasure to listen to.

Dr. Jane was in an appointment when I called, but she called me back within an hour. "First of all, let's do a brief summary of how cancer cells function. Cancer is actually a group of more than 100 diseases involving the uncontrolled division of cells. Hold on, this could be a long conversation. Have you had lunch yet, Papa Johnny?"

I told her I hadn't; I was much more interested in what she had to say than in lunch. However, if she hadn't had lunch, I would be happy take her out for lunch. She agreed to go out to lunch with me, and suggested I bring a notepad and a pen. I asked if I could bring a laptop and a tape recorder instead and she agreed.

A half hour later we settled into our booth for lunch at a wonderful Thai restaurant. After waiving off the server, I took out my laptop and tape recorder and told her to 'go to town.' She laughed and said I had better be careful what I asked for, this was a big passion of hers and she could go on forever. I laughed along with her and said I was ready for her. I really enjoyed talking and listening to Dr. Jane, she is incredibly knowledgeable and interesting.

"Okay, let's start out with some of the common characteristics of cancer cells. What everyone agrees on is that apoptosis, a normal genetic program in every cell, is turned off in cancer cells. Apoptosis is a preprogrammed death process that gets provoked by a number of different cellular situations, including the simple natural life-cycle of a cell. But with the genetic program turned off, the cells, now called cancer cells, simply keep replicating without any control and nothing dies.

Another common characteristic of various types of cancer cells is the cell membrane. Sugar can cross the membrane, but oxygen cannot. Without oxygen, the inside of a cancer cell becomes acidic. Cancer cells require a lot more sugar to produce the same amount of fuel, or ATP, as a normal cell. It was the 1931 Nobel Laureate, Otto Warburg, who recognized cancer cells have a very different energy metabolism than healthy cells. Huge amounts of sugars are fermented in the acidic cancer cell to produce the same amount of ATP. The by-product of producing ATP in cancer cells is lactic acid, which is sent to the liver. The sugar creates a low pH or acidic environment inside the cancer cells and the lactic acid creates a low pH in the liver. The more cancer there is, the lower the pH, the greater the general fatigue.

As I mentioned, the lactic acid is taken to the liver and the liver converts the lactic acid back into sugar or glucose. It requires a lot of energy and nutrients to make this conversion and it is also is hard on the liver. This is one of the reasons why many cancer patients actually die of liver cachexia, a wasting of the liver.

At that point she stopped long enough to catch the attention of our server. I paused my tape recording. Dr. Jane ordered a cup of tea and I ordered one too. She didn't order any lunch at that point, so I didn't either. She started up again with a passion and I turned the recorder back on.

"Another common characteristic is the tumor's capacity to provoke angiogenesis, which is the development of new blood vessels from which the cancer can extract a huge amount of nutrients from the body to keep growing.

What chemotherapy typically attempts to do is destroy the cancer's DNA so that it cannot reproduce. Unfortunately, this can only happen if the cancer cell is actually in a reproductive cycle.

Cancer cells grow really fast for a short period and then stop replicating for a longer period of time. If the clinician doesn't identify whether the cancer cells are in stage two of reproduction, the chemotherapy that is administered will harm every other cell in the body that is in growth cycle but have no effect on the cancer cell.

Now we know there are all kinds of compounds that can affect any one of these components."

I needed to clarify, "By components you mean, angiogenesis, apoptosis, and the cellular membrane? Did I miss anything?"

Dr. Jane smiled, "You're on your toes Papa Johnny. Well done.

Since we know cancer cells need a lot sugar, we know we need to restrict any sugars in the diet, both direct sugars, artificial sugars, and foods that turn into sugar."

"What do you mean foods that turn into sugar?" That was a new one for me.

"Simple carbs, foods like oranges, foods made with flours, all turn into sugars that are detrimental."

"What do mean oranges? I thought oranges were good for you."

"Yes, oranges used to be good for you. Most orange grove soils are depleted in magnesium. That affects both the fibers and the vitamin C in oranges. Consequently, most oranges tend to turn to sugar in the body."

"Wow, I didn't know that!"

"Getting back to cancer, the rationale is that if the cancer cells don't get the sugars they need, they cannot grow. However, if the cancer cells don't get the sugar they need from the diet, they steal it from 'normal' cells. So, getting sugar out of the diet is only part of the solution.

That is why we also have to stop the angiogenesis so that the cancer cells do not deplete the rest of the body.

Finally, we need to protect the liver from liver cachexia. We need to help the liver produce more glutathione to protect itself.

Glutathione is one of the key components the immune system requires to develop and respond to anything, including cancer. Unfortunately, many of the chemotherapies destroy glutathione which then prevents the body from destroying the cancer. Glutathione is involved in a *huge* number of other processes, but the really important ones relating to cancer include correcting DNA that has gone wrong in a new cell and/or destroying the new cancer cell, and of course, supporting the immune system so that it can also destroy the cancer cells. Are you aware that the average body makes about 1 million cancer cells a day? Glutathione and the immune system are responsible for keeping that under control.

Research shows some kinds of cancer cells can disguise themselves, so the immune system does not recognize that they need to destroy those cells. We have to use other methods, such as herbs and foods to:

- Alter the actual functioning of the cancer cell;
- Alter the cell membrane;
- Turn on the DNA of the cancer cells responsible for apoptosis;
- Block the angiogenesis; and
- Increase the glutathione levels.

There are a number of different treatment protocols we can work with.

Okay, that's enough for a moment. Let's order lunch."

I turned off the recorder and we decided to share a couple of dishes. The waitress came over to take our order and observed, "It looks like you guys are really getting deep into something heavy duty for lunch."

"You're right, but this gal is absolutely phenomenal, and she can cure the world of almost anything," I laughed with the waitress. She took our order and when she left I nodded to the recorder and Dr. Jane started again.

"First off, let me correct that statement. I cannot cure the body of everything. In fact, I can't cure anything."

I was stunned.

Hold on a minute. Wasn't she always curing all our family issues? "I don't follow. You are a physician. You have helped my extended family in so many ways. What do you mean, you don't cure anything?"

"Well I don't think I have the capacity to cure anything. Your body has a wisdom and knowledge that goes way beyond anything we know. We are only in the very beginning stages of understanding how and why the body does what it does. What we know is when we give the body various nutrients, the body knows what to do with them. We know when the body's natural healing processes get sidetracked, we can help the body eliminate the toxins and blockages preventing it from its natural healing processes and provide it with the nutrients it may be deficient in and we can help the Immune system regulate itself again.

We have a variety of ways of helping the body re-engage in its natural healing processes and that's what makes us so different from Western Conventional medicine. We don't attempt to manage the symptoms with artificial and/or synthetic drugs. We don't assume we know better than the body. We want to work with the body and enable it to do what it is supposed to do - eliminate the underlying issues causing the symptoms. Do you get that?"

I thought for a minute and summarized, "So I think what you are saying is that neither you nor MDs can heal the body. Your work is engaging the body in the processes it needs to engage in, in order to heal. In contrast, MDs provide artificial synthetic drugs to manage the symptoms rather than healing the body."

"Good, you got it. Well done."

I smiled and said, "Am I going to get an A?"

She laughed and suggested we get back to the topic of cancer. "Do you know one of the causes of cancer is chemotherapy? It's actually printed on the chemo drug warning labels. The chemotherapy may create a second kind of cancer in the body you didn't initially have! That's nuts. When people allow for surgical methods to draw out a piece of a tumor to determine if it is carcinogenic, that can also cause the cancer to spread.

There are all kinds of theories on what causes the different cancers and they may all be right. The theories include natural DNA dysfunction, depleted immune system, depleted glutathione, and pleomorphic bacteria that block the production of ATP. Do you know that the pleomorphic bacteria were discovered back in 1890?"

I shook my head no. I had seen something regarding it on the internet but hadn't followed through with it. "What are pleomorphic bacteria?"

"Okay, thanks for catching me, I try to remember to use language that everyone understands, but I sometimes slip up. Pleomorphic cells or organisms are the ones that can alter their shape or size in response to their environment."

"Wow, that's kind of neat, but how do you deal with them then?" it was a lot more complicated than I had thought.

"Well there are all kinds of methods of destroying these pleomorphic bacteria, I have looked at some of the equipment, but I don't actually use any of them. These devices are called things like the Quantum Pulse, Photon Genie, and High RF Frequency Protocol devices."

Dr. Jane directed me to some additional websites for further information, even if I didn't use it in the book. As I paid for lunch, she again offered to provide me whatever additional information I needed for my book. She was pleased with my chosen topic for the Book Club and was happy to provide whatever information might be of help to me.

I had to stop and think about how how our conversation compared with the MD I had tried to talk with. There was a huge difference in their tone and attitude, in their willingness to talk, and in their approach to healing the body. A world of difference.

Chapter 7

Depression

When I began writing this book, I decided to deal with each of the chapters a little differently. I might approach a different professional, for instance, whether I started with GP or an MD with a specialized field of interest. Or it might be whether I started with Conventional Western medicine or REAL medicine. It might be where I did my research, books or online, etc. For this chapter, I thought I would start with a psychiatrist.

I learned from the last time I went to an MD that if I wanted to talk with a specialist, I needed the MD to think I had a disorder, or dysfunction. So, I went to a clinic and claimed I was suffering from depression for some time. The MD recommended me to a psychiatrist and got an appointment for me.

Before I went to the appointment, I looked up the typical symptoms of someone with depression might suffer from and the medications they prescribed. I figured I was pretty prepared when I got to the psychiatrist's appointment.

I gave the usual profile of symptoms and he asked me a few questions about my life. He then gave me a prescription for Paxil. I asked him why he prescribed Paxil. He explained it was a good prescription for someone who suffered from depression. I explained I had read somewhere that research showed anti-depressants like Prozac, Zoloft and Paxil were no more effective than placebos.[59]

The psychiatrist wanted to know where I read that. As I had done my homework and was prepared, I provided him with a list of several different sites. He got rather agitated and explained he was the one with the education and either I followed his guidelines, or I could leave.

I asked him not to get upset with me. I really just wanted some information. I explained I wanted to learn about anti-depressants and wanted his help. He calmed down a bit and allowed me to ask questions. I explained my understanding was that depression was the result of low serotonin levels in the brain and asked if that was correct. He agreed that was right.

I asked if there was a test I could take to determine if I had low serotonin levels. He said they could analyze a blood sample but that usually they didn't. If they took blood tests, it was to rule out other things. Consequently, they usually went on the basis of symptoms the client presented.

I asked if he was aware of the different blood profiles for different types of depression. He didn't have a clue what I was talking about. I asked if he was aware of all the different physiological conditions that cause depression.[60]

He appeared frustrated and assumed I was challenging him. I tried to explain I just wanted more information but he wasn't willing to talk with me any further. Apparently, I already had more information than he did. I was shown the door.

I left the psychiatrist's office and went straight to the Gibson Clinic. The receptionist laughed when she saw me and asked if I wanted to take out a cot and make my stay permanent. I laughed with her and asked if Dr. Jim was in. Dr. Jim was a psychotherapist and so I thought he might be the best one to talk with. He was with a client and so I had to wait for a bit. I asked the receptionist if there was a computer I could use while I was waiting and there was. I wanted to have the material printed out for Dr. Jim in case he wasn't aware of it. After all, he didn't prescribe drugs.

Dr. Jim came into the conference room when he was finished with his client and as always, gave me a big hug. "Hi Papa Johnny, how are you? Are you here to learn or to get healthy?" he laughed.

"Well thanks to you guys, I am pretty healthy, so I guess I am here to learn by asking more questions. I just came from a psychiatrist's office. I asked him questions about depression. He got pretty frustrated with me and didn't want to talk, so I thought I would come and pick your brain instead."

"Well I do have another client coming in shortly, but I can give you 30 minutes. Fire away and we will see what we can do."

"Well first off; have you read the research showing all the different physiological conditions that cause depression?"

"Yes, I remember one that came out recently. If I remember correctly, they looked at about 2,800 patients and found in some it was an inability to make serotonin, or the reuptake of serotonin was too quick; some had problems with both impaired serotonin production and extreme oxidative stress.[61]

Now that didn't identify low glutathione levels as being the cause of the oxidative stress, but I would bet it was. For some, it was an inability to properly metabolize metals; in particular high copper levels which effected their dopamine and norepinephrine levels. The next group had to do with low levels of B vitamins. And the last group, showed toxic metal overload. I don't know if they tested for low levels of magnesium which has also been shown to cause depression. Did I get it right?"

"Yes, that is dead on. Why don't psychiatrists test for those things and what are you doing just talking with people if you know it can be the result of biochemistry?"

"Well, that's two questions, so let's start with the first one. More often than not, practitioners don't keep up with the research. They don't have the time, or they don't have the inclination, but for whatever their reasons, they just don't. But you know us natural health people; we are all about the current research. At least in this clinic.

The second question is more complex. First of all, there are a lot of issues that have to do with how people interpret and respond to the world: their underlying value systems, how they see themselves in the world, and how they deal with stress, frustration or decision making. As a practitioner, I do look at these issues. If these kinds of issues appear healthy, then we look for all the other kinds of issues.

And there are a number of other areas that may be contributing to the symptom profile. I have the clinic here with practitioners who deal with those issues like the oxidative stress, low levels of glutathione, and a depletion of minerals like magnesium. In addition, there are all kinds of concerns linked to depression: adrenal issues and liver issues as well as gut issues – specifically with imbalances in the gut microbiota. The individual and the symptoms they have determine the tests we run. Like anything else we have to be aware there are always a number of issues that can cause a similar symptom profile.

We also have to be aware that gut issues, for example, can control how we think, feel and behave. So even if we haven't run any kinds of biological or microbiological test, we want to know what the diet is like, what are the stressors like, how long have the stressors been going on, etc. That way we can know whether or not we need to run other tests.

If we are open and receptive and keen on the research, it helps us stay ahead of all the possibilities."

"So, if all of these things can cause depression, why are they allowed to simply dish out anti-depressants like candy?"

"You know the answer to that, Papa Johnny. It is a matter of who controls the information and what makes money. Who has the power and control? Big Pharma makes a billion dollars a day on any given anti-depressant and controls the information given to practitioners.

If people are willing to simply pay for ineffective drugs without doing any research themselves, they are in effect being controlled by Big Pharma. All very sad but true."

I thanked Dr Jim for his time and left the clinic feeling grateful for the information but deeply frustrated by the control Big Parma is exerting just to make money.

It filled me with righteous anger and made me feel slightly queasy.

I really wanted to get this book out there to show people what is really going on.

Chapter 8
Diabetes

I had listened to what the Gibsons had said during our potluck dinner and I knew another area to focus on was diabetes. So, in this chapter, I will share what I found easily researching good sources on the internet as recommended by the Gibsons.

It is general knowledge that sugar, insulin resistance and obesity cause diabetes, right?

Surprisingly, this is very incomplete!

Would you believe there are all kinds of other issues that can cause diabetes ranging from metal toxicity, to infections, to adrenal issues, to the microbiota in your gut?

Yes, metal toxicity has been shown to be part of the problem. Most of you will guess *mercury* is one of the metals, and you are right. Research has shown for years that mercury poisoning is associated with elevated levels of glucose in the urine. Whether organic, inorganic or elemental/metallic mercury, they all cause damage to the body at a cellular level. The types of affected cells include:

- Alveolar cells (cells lining the lungs)
- Astrocytes (a type of glial cell supporting the brain and spinal cord neurons)
- Epithelial cells (cells lining the lymph system and blood/vascular system)
- Gingival fibroblast cells (the stems cells found in the gums)
- Lymph cells (cells found in the lymphatic system)
- Renal cells (kidney cells)
- Pancreatic islet beta cells (cells producing insulin)

These types of cells all show a direct relationship to DNA and damaging oxidative stress aka free radicals. Unlike most metals, which are used by the body to varying extents, mercury has no know known use in the body. Any mercury, whether it is in the fillings of your teeth or from salmon or from vaccinations or any other source, causes direct damage to cells in a variety of ways. Further, it is very difficult for your body to eliminate mercury.

Arsenic is another toxin that can cause diabetes. I am an old fart, but surely you have heard of those murder mysteries where the victim is poisoned by arsenic. There is even a play and pretty good movie starring Cary Grant – *Arsenic and Old Lace.*

Did you know we get *arsenic* in our commercial chicken? Arsenic is also found in our plant soils and is readily taken up by many plants and crops such as rice.

Arsenic in our body can cause diabetes and other issues:

- Cancer
- Nervous system disorders
- Peripheral vascular disease
- Endocrine disruption
- Disrupt the processes regulating insulin resistance.

Have you heard of *cadmium*? It is highly toxic to the body. It accumulates in various organs and can cause massive damage.

- Accumulates in the liver (blocks organ tubules preventing reabsorption of calcium)
- Increases lipid (cholesterol) peroxidation
- Decreases insulin release
- Damages insulin receptors

On the other hand, unlike mercury the body does use cadmium, but only in minute doses.

So, having too much of some minerals can cause diabetes. The flip side of the coin is that deficiencies in essential trace minerals like **chromium** and **zinc** or a non-metal element like **selenium** can also cause dysfunctions in the body that provoke diabetic symptoms.

The gut *microbiota* can also provoke diabetic symptoms. Research shows if the good bacteria in our gut is either deficient OR if certain bacteria outnumber other ones, they also provoke diabetic symptoms and/or provoke issues such as:

- Alzheimer's
- Cholesterol issues
- Depression
- High blood pressure
- Non-alcoholic fatty liver disorders
- Obesity
- Parkinson's[62]

I was shocked to discover evidence indicating that maybe diabetes causes obesity as opposed to the other way around.

Most people who have diabetes, or know of a loved one with diabetes, have heard of the drug metformin. Did you know metformin is a man-made synthetic version of a plant compound called berberine? Plants with the natural compound in them can have a much more effective impact on your diabetes and can actually eliminate your diabetes.

The isolated synthetic berberine compound called metformin is less effective for a number of reasons. One of the most predominant side effects is the decrease in CoQ10 which is required by the mitochondria in the cells to make fuel.

I was surprised but pleased to discover that more and more physicians are daring to speak out against the 'old men's club' regarding previously believed causes of diabetes. Dr. Peter Attia believes we need to step out of the box and look at different possibilities when it comes to diabetes.[63]

It seems there is some hope after all. I was beginning to lose faith in Western Conventional medicine.

Chapter 9
What's left?

I could carry on and look at a variety of other diseases and disorders, though I don't think I am going to find anything different. So, I thought I needed to move down a different path.

I learned scientists have so many options to manipulate data it wasn't funny. However, research studies are predominantly controlled by whoever provides the funding. No matter what area of medicine I looked at, and granted I only looked at a few major areas, there was corruption, misleading information, negative results buried, and false positive results claimed that may have nothing to do with the actual results.

What about the actual politics going on? This was what I started out wanting to research. What I found was even more disturbing.

Joachim Hagopian wrote a very powerful article in Global Research titled *The Evils of Big Pharma Exposed*. He explains the politics very well.

...Big Pharma seeks enormous profits over the health and well-being of the humans it serves...the story of Big Pharma is the exact same story of how Big Government, Big Oil, and Big Agri-Chemical Giants like Monsanto have come to power. The controlling shareholders of all these major industries are one and the same.[64]

These are a few European and the US 'oligarch families' who worked towards eliminating competition behind the façade of 'free enterprise'.

The net profit for 2012, amongst the top eleven, amounted to $85 billion in just that one year.[65]

That kind of money wields a lot of power.

One of the major families, the Rockefellers, privatized healthcare in the US and has financed and have played a big role in healthcare and Big Pharma since the 1930s.

Bottom line, if humans are healthy, the healthcare industry does not survive. Thus, it's in its own inherently self-serving interest to promote illness in the name of wellness.[66]

I highly recommend you read the full article.

I knew about Venn diagrams before, but seeing them explained, I understood the overlap between government and Big Pharma and found it disturbing. The following Venn diagram illustrates the overlap of members of the US Federal Government who have also represented Big Pharma since 2011.

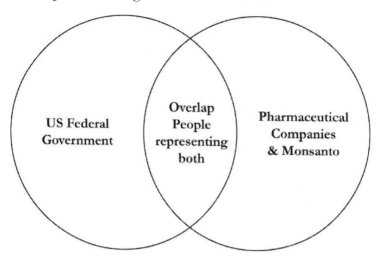

There are actually 19 different Venn Diagrams showing just how invested members of government are in big business. As opposed to representing the people, they represent companies like GE, Media, Monsanto, Goldman Sachs, Comcast, Big Oil, etc.[67]

When it comes to the finances, I already learned that Big Pharma didn't have any moral or ethical obligation to our health. But it does have a legal responsibility to making money for the shareholders.

I think Joachim Hagopian said it very well:

Also because natural healing substances cannot be patented, Big Pharma has done its sinister best to squelch any and all knowledge and information that come from the far more affordable means of alternative health sources that explore ancient traditional cultures' medicinal use of hemp along with thousands of other plants and roots that could threaten drug profits and power of Big Pharma and modern medicine as they're currently practiced and monopolized.[68]

But there are other problems too. The US court system has made it almost financially impossible for anyone to make a claim against Big Pharma. In addition, to make a claim, there is a minimum required number of individuals that need to band together. Then they need to find a lawyer that is actually willing to stand up to Big Pharma. Then, despite the fact that Big Pharma provides precious little accurate information on how and why a given drug works, the law suit is required to provide phenomenal evidence the drug actually caused harm.

All in all, it is made an incredibly expensive and difficult process to undertake. One of the reasons the process is difficult is because the system favors the status quo. So, if the FDA already approved a drug, you are going to have a difficult time going against the existing research, no matter how flawed it is and the accepted belief system.

In addition, US judges have "gate keeping authority" that allows them the right to reject what they perceive to be evidence threatening the accepted medical belief systems. They are encouraged to support the status quo.

Further, the government not only protects Big Pharma but will bail them out when necessary.

> The truth is the US government will knuckle under to Big Pharma, Wall Street and Big Banks every single time, even when it knows these "too big to fail" criminals repeatedly violate laws intended to protect the public. And constantly bailing them out at overburdened taxpayer expense only causes them to become more brazenly criminal, knowing they will always be protected by their co-conspirators the feds.[69]

Another problem the physicians and the patients are up against is that even when there is evidence that a drug is ineffective and dangerous, it can remain on the market! Just because it harmed (or even killed) one person, doesn't mean it is harmful to the majority or even a minority.

In Chapter 4, we explored how Big Pharma has the money to create perceptions of safety and efficacy, even when there isn't any. These false perceptions are directed to both the general public as well as physicians, academic opinion leaders and scientists. Once those perceptions become accepted and widespread, we now have a standard of care that is very difficult to fight.

I started to wonder if the general rule of thumb for Big Pharma, is to continue with false advertising until they get caught.

I shared this disturbing thought with Mary.

Mary said, "That's a pretty heavy statement to make. How do you prove something like that?"

"Well, look at the process they go through. When they are caught, they are 'punished' with fines, which sounds good on the surface until you start looking at the fines, they are just a slap on the wrist for them. They may have to pay out millions of dollars for fraud, fraudulent campaigns, product liability, ghostwriting, bribing, etc., but when a given drug makes over a billion dollars a day, these fines are merely a drop in the bucket and do nothing to change their policies.

In addition, we have to look at how much of the media is controlled by Big Pharma. The media is hugely dependent on Big Pharma marketing funds. Thus, impartial journalism about Big Pharma is pushed to the side and false advertising is allowed to prevail, to protect the incoming dollars to the media corporation.

Commercials fund cable television and if you watch television you have surely seen those super long commercials for pharmaceuticals. Marketing is all about making you believe you have a *need* for something. These commercials start with a story of either how the drug saved someone or how the drug could have saved someone, or drastically improved their lives. They quickly provide a long list of issues that prevent you from taking the drug, then provide an even longer list of the side effects you might experience, including death, if you take the drug. The final segment tells you how beneficial the drug might be as if none of the prior information was of any value. The final statement tells you to 'ask your doctor if the drug is right for you'.

We are being bombarded with these messages continuously through all types of advertising. I used to listen to the advertisements wondering which drug would be best for me. Now I just get angry when they come on.

While we would like to believe scientists in the universities operate with a different perspective, it turns out too many of them don't. The universities push for grants and donations from Big Pharma and many are very dependent on Big Pharma money. So, the individual professor is 'incentivised' to cooperate in order to keep the university's funding and Big Pharma is given a tremendous amount of leeway in controlling the design, analysis, etc. of the given study."

In frustration, I went for a walk with Mary to clear my head before I went back to the computer and continued my exploration.

The research I found revealed that false premises or beliefs are perpetuated and become more ingrained over time, not only with the general public, but also with the practitioners and the scientists.

The whole Cholesterol Myth, and need for statin drugs, is a good example of how a falsehood can be perpetuated. Another falsehood is that low serotonin levels cause depression, which requires an anti-depressant drug. This hypothesis has never proven. Claims that we cannot eliminate arthritis, or diabetes, or dementia, or umpteen other conditions are also false.

The false premises result in physicians prescribing drugs for a person's lifetime. There are too many examples of false premises prevailing despite loads of studies and evidence to the contrary.

Similar kinds of studies also show it takes upwards of 40 years for good research to get to the physician and to the hospitals. I wonder who prevents the information from becoming wide spread. It is obviously not in the best financial interest of Big Pharma to allow marketing of simple, inexpensive ways to eliminate conditions, when they can make billions of dollars daily by marketing and creating a perceived need for continued pharmaceuticals.

We certainly cannot depend on the FDA to protect us. The best they can do is to allow drugs, whose limited published research shows positive results indicating a high established level of safety and efficacy, or to eliminate drugs that don't live up to their claims. Unfortunately, removing the ineffective drugs or drugs that cause huge issues (like death), take a long time to remove.

To make matters worse, the FDA is partially funded by Big Pharma, through the Prescription Drug User Fee Act (PDUFA). Further, their various approval boards and advisory committees are made up of people who are also on the Big Pharma payroll, so whether anything is given approval, or not, by the FDA really means nothing. Further, a panel of 200 experts that established the guidelines with the FDA, revealed one third of the panel had financial interest in the drugs they considered.[70]

Another example, provided in the same source, was taken from 2004 when the National Cholesterol Education Program called for sharply lowering the desired levels of "bad" cholesterol. It was revealed eight of the nine members of the panel writing the recommendations had financial ties to the makers of cholesterol-lowering drugs.[71]

To add insult to injury, the FDA has a pre-emption policy banning private lawsuits suing Big Pharma in state courts after a drug label has been approved by the FDA!!![72]

A really good article, *Attorney Tells All: How the U.S. Courts Shield Big Pharma from Liability*, peopleschemist.com interviews one of the top lawyers who fights Big Pharma and is worth reading.[73]

In recent years, MDs are not exempt from accountability. There are apparently a number of lawsuits against Big Pharma for paying physicians to push "off-label" uses of drugs. Off-label means using the drugs to manage symptoms for issues that research has never addressed. ProPublica.org identifies several whistleblowers, lawsuits and settlements made because of Big Pharma's illegal use of funds to manipulate physicians.[74]

A terrific article entitled, *Death by Medicine*, was written by Gary Null, PhD, Carolyn Dean, MD and ND, Martin Feldman, MD, Debora Rasio, MD, and Dorothy Smith, PhD. There is both a short and a long version of the article that I recommend you read.[75]

The long article provides a lot of very interesting information. It states, "Approximately 7.5 million unnecessary medical and surgical procedures are performed annually in the US, while approximately 8.9 million Americans are hospitalized unnecessarily."[76]

The statistics they provide for August of 2006 show the medical system, including physicians, hospitals and drugs, cause 783,936 deaths a year, costing about $282 billion. Consequently, they state "Nearly 800,000 Americans die each year at the hands of government-sanctioned medicine, while the FDA and other government agencies pretend to protect the public by harassing those who offer safe alternatives."[77]

I couldn't find more current statistics that were not laced with "gross inaccuracies" even the World Health Organization made the following statement:

Countries continue to invest in their national cause-of-death information systems, but the gross inaccuracies in the data render them unsuitable for accurately describing the countries' main health problems or their burden of disease.[78]

It seems Big Pharma has learned to cover its tracks.

They also provide comparative numbers. During the same time period, about 700,000 died of heart disease and about 550,000 died of cancer. Obviously, the American medical system is the number one killer.

I don't know about you, but that really threw me. The very system that is supposed to protect and help us is actually robbing us blind, while killing us! An article in the Washingtonblog.com concluded with:

> "And we've previously documented that the government sometimes uses raw power to **cover up corruption in the medical and scientific fields.**
>
> Postscript: Corruption is not limited to the medical or scientific fields. Instead, corruption has become systemic throughout every profession … and is so pervasive that it is **destroying the very fabric of America.**"[79] [70]

So, what are we going to do?

I had to laugh, when I said to Mary, "I will certainly never simply trust anything an MD tells me again. I will research everything he/she prescribes and always look up the law suits and conflicts."

She responded with, "Well it is our body, I guess we should take responsibility for it and not just hand it away to someone else."

No kidding. I had never thought of it that way. Perhaps more importantly, I will always make sure I go to people like the Gibson practitioners, people who want to sit down and take the time with me, people who are on top of the research, people who want to identify and eliminate the underlying problem as opposed to those who are trained to simply manage the symptoms with synthetic drugs, which are at best questionable, and we know they deplete the body of nutrients and cause so many additional problems.

What are **you** going to do?

References

1. Siu AL, Sonnenberg FA, Manning WG, et al. Inappropriate use of hospitals in a randomized trial of health insurance plans. N Engl J Med. 1986 Nov 13;315(20):1259-66.

2. Siu AL, Manning WG, Benjamin B. Patient, provider and hospital characteristics associated with inappropriate hospitalization. Am J Public Health. 1990 Oct;80(10):1253-6.

3. Eriksen BO, Kristiansen IS, Nord E, et al. The cost of inappropriate admissions: a study of health benefits and resource utilization in a department of internal medicine. J Intern Med. 1999 Oct;246(4):379-87.

Members of the Entwined Book Project

The following is a list of the characters and the books they plan to write or have written

Smiths: Married for 23 yrs at the age of 24 & 25, October 25

Name: Maria, 47
Book: A Love that Crosses Time
Issue: Adrenal Fatigue
Character: Realtor that is a go getter, but family is most important; loves husband dearly

Name: Duncan, 48
Book: A Book for Men: How to Create a Good Marriage
Issue: Enlarged left ventricle
Character: Devoted husband and father

Name: Jessie, 20, daughter
Book: Female Sexuality
Issue: Diabetes
Character: University student, initially wants to be an MD but moves into Real Medicine, boyfriend Steve

Name: Jasmine, 15, daughter
Book: A Time Travel Romance
Issue: Asthma
Character: Dancer, somewhat shy, boyfriend Nick

Name: John, 9, son
Book: How Aliens Would Interpret our Planet
Issue: Allergies
Character: Artist, loves Granddad

Friends
Name: Steve, 20, Jessie's boyfriend
Book: How to Deal with Alcoholic Husbands
Issue: Alcoholic father
Character: University student, father alcoholic, submissive mother, avoids homelife, loves the Smith family

Name: Nick, 15, Jasmine's boyfriend
Book: Music, Sound & Other Energies for Healing
Character: Dancer, somewhat shy, Steve is like an older brother

Maria's Parents
Name: Grandma Mary
Book: Manage or Eliminate Arthritis
Issue: Arthritis
Character: Sweet; grandma type; adores grandpa

Name: Papa Johnny
Book: The Politics of Health
Issue: Dementia
Character: Funny old guy; set in his ways, but changing his mind

Maria's sister Carol and family
Name: Carol, Maria's sister
Book: Emotional Eating
Issue: Weight
Character: Kinda of belligerent; but wants the best for her family
Husband George

Name: George, Maria's brother-in-law
Book: Covering Up Suicidal Thinking
Issue: Depression
Character: He's tries to be the man; but really isn't; not confident like Duncan; but holds his own
With his wife Carol

Name: Tim, 19, Maria's nephew
Book: What it Feels Like NOT to be Understood
Issue: Paranoia
Character: Weak; not well developed; insecure, girlfriend Shelley

Name: Sherry, 15, Maria's niece
Book: A Romance About Gaining Self Control
Issue: Obsessive-Compulsive
Character: Struggles with control issues, boyfriend Randy

Name: Shelley
Book: Teen Age Empowerment
Issue:
Character: Tim's girlfriend

Maria's brother Dave and family
Name: Dave, Maria's brother
Book: When Enough is Enough
Issue: Divorce
Character: Dave compassionate man; gives too much;
finally divorced bipolar abusive Joan

Grandma Mary's brother and family
Name: Dan
Book: How to Design Your Dream Home
Issue: High cholesterol, hyper -tension
Character: He's a good guy; but private; hasn't dated
anyone since his wife Judy died years ago

Gibson family – own the Gibsons Clinic
Name: Dr Jim
Book: Personality Styles & Marriage
Issue:
Character: Psychotherapist Social/outgoing; fun but
wise, Julie's husband

Name: Julie
Book: A Book comparing East & West Religious
Philosophies
Issue:
Character: Physiotherapist, gentle; sweetheart;
nurturing, Jim's wife

Name: Dr Jane
Book: A New Integrative Model for Cellular Healing
Issue:
Character: Dr of Natural Medicine Academic; knows
her stuff; confident in her knowledge
Gibson's daughter

Name: Dr Daniel
Book: A Very Unique Cookbook
Issue:
Character: PhD Nutrition, academic but has fun with food,
Gibson's son

Name: Nanny Sarah
Book: Romance and Cerebral Palsy
Issue:
Character: Acupuncturist, gentle, nurturing, mothering, accommodating, Jim's mother

Name: Pappy
Book: Eliminating Autism
Issue:
Character: Master Herbalist, fun, happy go lucky, loves life, Jim's father

Endnotes

[1]http://www.thelancet.com/pdfs/journals/lancet/PIIS 0140-6736(15)60696-1.pdf

[2]http://www.nybooks.com/articles/2009/01/15/drug-companies-doctorsa-story-of-corruption/

[3]http://www.nybooks.com/articles/2009/01/15/drug-companies-doctorsa-story-of-corruption/

[4]http://www.thelancet.com/pdfs/journals/lancet/PIIS 0140-6736%2815%2960696-1.pdf

[5]http://www.macleans.ca/society/life/when-science-isnt-science-based-in-class-with-dr-john-ioannidis/

[6]http://www.sizediversityandhealth.org/images/uploaded/lies-damned-lies.pdf

[7]http://jama.jamanetwork.com/article.aspx?articleid=201218

[8] https://www.newscientist.com/article/dn3781-research-funded-by-drug-companies-is-biased/

[9]http://www.thelancet.com/pdfs/journals/lancet/PIIS 0140-6736%2815%2960696-1.pdf

10 http://www.macleans.ca/society/life/when-science-isnt-science-based-in-class-with-dr-john-ioannidis/

11http://www.theatlantic.com/magazine/archive/2010/11/lies-damned-lies-and-medical-science/308269/

12http://www.theguardian.com/science/2012/oct/01/tenfold-increase-science-paper-retracted-fraud

13http://link.springer.com/article/10.1007%2Fs11948-015-9668-7#/page-1

14 http://www.statnews.com/2015/12/13/clinical-trials-investigation/

15http://www.sizediversityandhealth.org/images/uploaded/lies-damned-lies.pdf

16http://www.bumc.bu.edu/crro/files/2010/01/Colton-2-21-07.pdf

17https://blogs.bournemouth.ac.uk/research/2016/01/11/ref-review-to-be-led-by-lord-stern-of-brentford/

18http://www.thelancet.com/pdfs/journals/lancet/PIIS0140-6736(15)60696-1.pdf

19 http://www.raps.org/Regulatory-Focus/News/2014/08/11/20005/Number-of-Drug-Recalls-Surges-at-FDA-Led-by-Mid-Level-Concerns/

20 https://www.statista.com/statistics/618383/total-fda-drug-enforcement-reports

[21]http://jama.jamanetwork.com/article.aspx?articleid= 209653

[22] http://www.ncbi.nlm.nih.gov/pubmed/16014596

[23]http://www.ncbi.nlm.nih.gov/pmc/articles/PMC370 0330/

[24] http://www.kevinmd.com/blog/2014/04/negative-results-clinical-trials-reported.html

[25]http://www.californiahealthline.org/articles/2010/11 /18/propublica-disciplined-doctors-receiving-drug-company-funding

[26]http://www.theatlantic.com/magazine/archive/2010 /11/lies-damned-lies-and-medical-science/308269

[27] http://www.ncbi.nlm.nih.gov/pubmed/19588353

[28]https://proteinpower.com/drmike/2013/12/30/abs olute-risk-versus-relative-risk-need-know-difference/

[29]http://scienceblog.cancerresearchuk.org/2013/03/15 /absolute-versus-relative-risk-making-sense-of-media-stories/

[30] http://patient.info/health/absolute-risk-and-relative-risk

[31] www.drrosedale.com/videos#axzz3vjkKis5l Video titled: *Dr. Rosedale Exposing the Cholesterol Myth: Cholesterol is not the major culprit in heart disease*

32https://articles.mercola.com/sites/articles/archive/2011/10/22/debunking-the-science-behind-lowering-cholesterol-levels.aspx

33 http://www.sott.net/article/242516-Heart-surgeon-speaks-out-on-what-really-causes-heart-disease

34 http://www.sott.net/article/242516-Heart-surgeon-speaks-out-on-what-really-causes-heart-disease

35 http://www.sott.net/article/242516-Heart-surgeon-speaks-out-on-what-really-causes-heart-disease

36 http://www.sott.net/article/242516-Heart-surgeon-speaks-out-on-what-really-causes-heart-disease

37 http://www.bmj.com/content/347/bmj.f7267

38https://pharmacy.ucsf.edu/news/2012/08/conflicts-interest-significantly-underreported-systematic-reviews-drug-efficacy-safety

39http://www.sizediversityandhealth.org/images/uploaded/lies-damned-lies.pdf

40http://articles.mercola.com/sites/articles/archive/2011/10/15/mayo-clinic-finds-massive-fraud-in-cancer-research.aspx

41http://articles.mercola.com/sites/articles/archive/2011/10/15/mayo-clinic-finds-massive-fraud-in-cancer-research.aspx

42http://www.pnc.com.au/~cafmr/online/research/cancer.html

[43]https://paulingblog.wordpress.com/2008/10/28/clarifying-three-widespread-quotes/

[44] http://www.watbezieltons.nu/index.php/most-cancer-research-is-a-fraud/?lang=en

[45] http://www.watbezieltons.nu/index.php/most-cancer-research-is-a-fraud/?lang=en

[46]http://www.nature.com/nature/journal/v483/n7391/full/483531a.html

[47] http://www.watbezieltons.nu/index.php/most-cancer-research-is-a-fraud/?lang=en

[48]http://www.nature.com/nature/journal/v483/n7391/full/483531a.html

[49]http://vivisectionresearch.ca/Cancer%20Research%20a%20Super%20Fraud.pdf

[50] https://www.rense.com/general9/cre.htm

[51] https://www.cnbc.com/2019/02/11/this-is-the-real-reason-most-americans-file-for-bankruptcy.html

[52] https://www.bbc.com/news/business-28212223

[53] https://qz.com/1075285/new-data-show-that-cancer-drugs-cost-less-to-make-than-big-pharma-has-claimed/

[54] https://www.bbc.com/news/business-28212223

[55] http://www.dailymail.co.uk/health/article-2806496/War-cancer-stalling-pharmaceutical-firms-

create-drugs-know-make-profit-leading-scientist-claims.html

[56] Fourchalk, Holly, PhD. DNM® RHT. *Cancer: Why want you don't know about your treatment could harm you.* Summer Bay Press. Vancouver, BC. 2012.

[57] Walker, Morton, D.P.M. *Natural cancer remedies…! How you can defeat cancer without chemotherapy or surgery.* Online Publishing and Marketing LLC. USA. 2009.

[58] McKinney, Neil BSc. ND. *Naturopathic oncology: an encyclopedic guide for patients and physicians.* 2nd edition, Liaison Press. Vancouver, BC. 2012.

[59]http://www.sizediversityandhealth.org/images/uploaded/lies-damned-lies.pdf

[60]https://www.ncbi.nlm.nih.gov/pmc/articles/PMC3527816/

[61] https://www.foxnews.com/health/new-blood-urine-tests-find-5-distinct-types-of-depression-researcher-says

[62]http://www.tandfonline.com/doi/abs/10.4161/isl.1.3.9262

[63] http://blog.ted.com/why-our-understanding-of-obesity-and-diabetes-may-be-wrong-a-qa-with-surgeon-peter-attia

[64] http://www.globalresearch.ca/the-evils-of-big-pharma-exposed/5425382

65 http://www.globalresearch.ca/the-evils-of-big-pharma-exposed/5425382

66 http://www.globalresearch.ca/the-evils-of-big-pharma-exposed/5425382

67 https://www.geke.us/VennDiagrams.html

68 http://www.globalresearch.ca/the-evils-of-big-pharma-exposed/5425382

69 http://www.globalresearch.ca/the-evils-of-big-pharma-exposed/5425382

70http://www.nybooks.com/articles/2009/01/15/drug-companies-doctorsa-story-of-corruption/

71http://www.nybooks.com/articles/2009/01/15/drug-companies-doctorsa-story-of-corruption/

72 http://www.counterpunch.org/2007/01/10/how-the-fda-protects-big-pharma/

73 https://thepeopleschemist.com/attorney-interview-how-us-courts-shield-big-pharma/

74 http://www.propublica.org/article/lawsuits-say-pharma-illegally-paid-doctors-to-push-their-drugs

75 The short version is found at www.webdc.com/pdfs/deathbymedicine.pdf and the longer version is found at www.lifeextension.com/magazine/2006/8/report_death/Page-01

[76]http://www.lifeextension.com/magazine/2006/8/report_death/page-01

[77]http://www.lifeextension.com/magazine/2006/8/report_death/page-01

[78] https://www.who.int/bulletin/volumes/92/1/13-134106/en/

[79]

http://www.washingtonsblog.com/2015/06/editors-in-chief-of-worlds-most-prestigious-medical-journals-much-of-the-scientific-literature-perhaps-half-may-simply-be-untrue-it-is-simply-no-longer-poss.html

Manufactured by Amazon.ca
Bolton, ON

28790449R00094